DISEASES AND PARASITES OF DOGS AND CATS

DISEASES AND PARASITES OF DOGS AND CATS

Editor
Gove Hambidge

2016
BIOTECH BOOKS
Delhi - 1100 035

ISBN 81-7622-089-2

Original Title: Livestock Yearbook of Agriculture, 1942

Published by : **BIOTECH BOOKS**
1123/74, Tri Nagar,
Delhi - 110 035
Phone: 27382765
e-mail: biotechbooks@yahoo.co.in

Showroom : 4762-63/23, Ansari Road, Darya Ganj,
NEW DELHI - 110 002
Phone: 23245578, 23244987

Laser Typesetting : **Classic Computer Services**
Delhi - 110 035

Printed at : **Chawla Offset Printers**
Delhi - 110 052

PRINTED IN INDIA

CONTENTS

INTRODUCTION

Rabies and Its Control

Rabies can be controlled and even eradicated, but in the United States, which has so successfully combated other animal diseases, it is allowed to be widely prevalent.

The disease is caused by a virus, which attacks the brain and spinal cord, with fatal results. In this country it is spread chiefly by the bites of mad dogs; the virus exists in the animal's saliva and infects the wound. It has been estimated that about 15 per cent of the human beings bitten by mad dogs contract the disease unless they receive treatment, which consists of a series of vaccine injections. Among domestic animals, about 35 per cent of those bitten become infected. These are general figures only and have been estimated over a period of years. The incidence of the disease may be higher or lower in specific outbreaks.

In most cases, symptoms of the disease develop within 2 weeks to 3 months after infection. When a human being is bitten by a dog that might possibly be rabid, it is important to confine the animal under the observation of a veterinarian until the disease, if it is present, has a chance to develop and run its course. Death occurs within a few days after symptoms appear, and the dog's brain can then be examined for specific evidence of rabies. The treatment given to exposed human beings depends to a large extent on this evidence.

The symptoms of rabies in dogs follow two general patterns, the furious and the dumb forms, and both are described by Schoening in some detail. He also describes the symptoms in cats and in cattle. Many wild animals are subject to the disease; in 1940 there was a serious outbreak among foxes in several Southern States, centering in Georgia, during which at least 90 head of livestock contracted rabies from fox bites, and 17 human beings were given treatment. Schoening gives figures showing all the reported cases of rabies in each State during 1938 and 1939, including human beings, dogs, and all other animals, and briefly discusses the situation in other countries, showing that several have been free of this disease for the past 10 years.

The Pasteur treatment and its modifications are used after exposure to the disease. About 20 years ago a one-shot vaccine was developed to be used for dogs as a preventive before exposure. Although this vaccination has definite value, it can not be relied on as the sole method of controlling the disease, because there are dogs to which it does not give sure protection against a severe exposure. Moreover, the stray dog always plays an important part in the spread of the disease.

Adequate control or eradication of rabies demands the simultaneous use of several measures under uniform regulations applied by all States. Schoening quotes the 1939 and 1940 reports of the Committee on Rabies of the United States Live Stock Sanitary Association as, embodying a suitable programme for this country. In brief the regulations recommended are:

(1) Licence all dogs annually.

(2) Require that the dog wear the licence attached to its collar at all times when on public property.

(3) Destroy or impound all unlicensed dogs. Local conditions should determine whether impounded dogs can be safely returned to their owners or sold.

(4) Provide a sufficient full-time personnel to control stray and unlicensed dogs.

(5) Determine adequately whether any suspected dog is rabid. If it is, destroy all dogs that have been bitten or exposed, or quarantine them for 6 months on the owners' premises, or give the vaccination treatments and quarantine them for 2 months. In addition, place a 60-day quarantine on the entire area over which the rabid dog may have strayed, allowing no dog on public property during this period unless it is held on a leash not over 6 feet long in the hands of a competent person.

(6) Make ample funds available in each community for carrying out the regulations.

(7) Have the veterinary profession represented in the personnel concerned with the control of the disease and provide for adequate publicity in case of outbreaks and quarantines.

(8) Encourage or advocate preventive vaccination on a voluntary basis when it seems advisable, but do not give vaccinated dogs special privileges.

Distemper of Dogs

Distemper, "the scourge of dogdom," is quite similar to influenza in human beings and, like the latter, is caused primarily by a virus, followed by a secondary bacterial invasion. For the most part it attacks, young dogs from 2 months to a year old, producing a catarrhal, inflammation of all the mucous membranes of the body, frequently accompanied by nervous symptoms caused by disturbances of the brain and spinal cord. The disease is highly contagious and often fatal; affected animals should be promptly isolated, and the premises should be thoroughly disinfected.

Stein emphasizes that diagnosis and the prescription of treatment should be in the hands of a competent veterinarian. There is no cure, but injections of an antiserum administered early enough can lessen the severity of an attack. Otherwise, treatment consists in careful nursing and feeding.

Two basic methods of immunization are effective in preventing the disease, one involving the use of a vaccine and a living virus, the other the use of an antiserum and a living virus. Some investigators believe that puppies vaccinated under 4 to 6 months of age do not become completely immune; hence they should not be vaccinated until after this age. In case of imminent exposure, however, puppies 6 to 8 weeks old can be protected by a vaccine or antiserum and then immunized later.

Feline Enteritis

Considered to be the most serious disease of cats and frequently occurring in severe outbreaks, feline enteritis is especially disastrous to young animals, among which the mortality rate is often higher than 80 percent. The virus that causes the disease is spread by direct or indirect contact and by fleas. Stein describes the disease as sudden in its appearance and rapid and violent in its course, producing a high fever, an acute inflammation of the intestinal tract a marked decrease in the number of white blood cells, great depression, and rapid loss of flesh. Sometimes kittens die before any apparent symptoms develop. Parasitic infestation, undernourishment, and other devitalizing factors lower the resistance of animals.

Reports indicate that certain biological products-vaccines, antisera, and bacterins–are of value in combating feline enteritis, some being used as preventives and others to furnish temporary immunity or, in the early stages of the disease, to reduce the violence of its course. The administration of these products, or of drugs, should be undertaken only by a veterinarian. Affected cats should be immediately isolated, kept is warm dry quarters, and fed broth, milk, and raw eggs if they will take nourishment. It is important to disinfect the quarters thoroughly and to eliminate fleas.

Miscellaneous Diseases of Dogs and Cats

In a condensed account of a great many diseases and other conditions of dogs and cats, Stein gives general information and suggestions rather than details because of space limitations. This brief summary can do little more than list the topics he covers. As the author points out, even an elementary knowledge will help pet owners to keep their animals in good condition. For definite diagnosis and treatment it is necessary in most cases to consult a veterinarian specializing in the diseases of pets.

Abnormal growths or swellings encountered in pets include abscesses, cysts, tumors (malignant and nonmalignant), mumps, goiter, enlargements of the lymph glands caused by Hodgkins disease, and rupture (hernia).

Anal gland infection, followed by clogging of the glands, is especially likely to occur in old dogs.

Ascites (*dropsy*) is usually the result of diseases of the heart, liver, or kidneys.

Ailments of aged dogs include a considerable number of afflictions, some of which may require persistent treatment as well as good care and feeding.

Diseases of the digestive system are common in dogs and cats and are usually due to improper feeding. Various treatments are required according to the nature of the disturbance.

Depraved appetite (pica) may be due to nutritional deficiencies, parasites, or simply habit.

Foreign bodies sometimes lodge in the digestive tract and are likely to require veterinary attention. Regular grooming of cats will prevent their swallowing enough hair to form hair balls in the intestine.

Intestinal obstruction, caused by indigestible material, is likely to require irrigation and other special treatment.

Gastroenteritis, or intestinal inflammation, is a common ailment, especially of dogs, and is due to any one of a number of causes, including faulty feeding.

Hemorrhagic gastroenteritis, an inflammation accompanied by internal hemorrhage, is especially serious and demands veterinary attention.

Ear diseases include external and internal canker and a sensitive swelling called haemotoma, caused by an injury that ruptures small blood vessels.

Eclampsia, a nervous malady of nursing bitches, characterized by convulsions, is usually treated with injections of calcium gluconate.

Eye diseases include conjunctivitis, keratitis, ulcers on the cornea, cataract, glaucoma, and two types of eyelid affections known as entropion and ectropion.

Fits, characterized by convulsions and nervous spasms, are symptoms of some underlying disorder that may have any one of a number of causes. The cause must be determined to prevent further attacks.

Icterus (jaundice) may be a symptom of a liver disease or a stomach disorder, or it may be caused by a specific infection, considered to be identical with that responsible for Weil's disease in human beings.

Metritis and pyometra are diseases of the uterus due to various causes; severe cases require surgery.

Postrrior paralysis, or paralysis of the hindquarters, is due to any one of a considerable number of causes.

Urinary calculi, or stones in the kidney, bladder, or urethra, usually require surgical treatment.

Respiratory affections to which pet animals are subject include colds, laryngitis, bronchitis, pleurisy, and pneumonia.

Warts (*papilloma*) may be hard or soft, and certain types are considered to be contagious.

Poisoning demands immediate veterinary attention as well as first aid. The author deals with poisoning by arsenic, phosphorus, lead, strychnin, carbolic acid, carbon monoxide, snake bites, and decayed food.

Car sickness, not uncommon in nervous dogs, may be forestalled to some extent by certain simple precautions.

First aid is often required for pet animals; Stein tells what to do for some of the common injuries.

Spaying and castration of dogs and cats are briefly discussed by the author, with recommendations as to the best ages at which to have the operations performed.

Internal Parasites of Dogs and Cats

Price and Harwood discuss preventive measures and medicinal treatment at the end of their article, but in this brief summary prevention and treatment will be considered with the discussion of the parasites. As these authors point out, preventive measures are often not feasible on the farm, where dogs and cats usually run free. Medicinal treatment, they emphasize, should always be based on accurate diagnosis, which usually. requires expert knowledge. They argue against the periodical dosing of pet animals regardless of the presence of parasites; worm medicines are toxic and should be used only when necessary. They also stress the importance of good nutrition as a factor in building general resistance to internal parasites.

Protozoa

Minute one-celled organisms, of which two types cause important diseases in this country:

(1) *Piroplasmosis*: A *Piroplasma*, transmitted by the bite of ticks, attacks the red blood cells of dogs, causing an acute or chronic disease with symptoms that in some ways resemble those of distemper. *Prevention*: Control of ticks. *Medicinal treatment*: Injections of acaprin or other drugs.

(2) *Coccidiosis*: Caused by coccidia invading the intestinal tract, and transmitted by oocysts (egglike forms) passed in the foeces and contaminating the ground. Diarrhoea is the chief symptom in heavy infections. *Prevention*: Sanitation and prompt disposal of feces. *Medicinal treatment*: None available.

Flukes

The most important is the salmon-poisoning fluke, associated with a serious disease of dogs in the Pacific Northwest. This fluke passes part of its life cycle in a snail, another part in a salmonoid fish. Dogs acquire the parasite by eating the infected fish. Apparently a virus accompanies the fluke infestation in the intestines, causing a disease that resembles distemper and is fatal in 50 to 90 per cent of the untreated cases. *Prevention*: Keep raw fish away from dogs and cats. *Treatment*: Sulfanilamide (first used for this purpose in 1938).

Taperworms

(1) Several kinds of armed tapeworms (equipped with suckers and hooks) infest dogs, one kind infests cats, and at least two kinds infest both. The larvae (bladder worms) of these parasites develop in other mammals, including rodents, rabbits, hares, sheep, goats, cattle, swine, and in at least one case, human beings; one armed tapeworm, however, usually passes its larval stages in certain fleas and lice. Mild infestations in dogs and cats apparently do no harm; heavy ones may result in such symptoms as digestive disturbances and general restlessness. *Prevention*: Control fleas and lice; do not permit dogs and cats to feed on the infected fresh of intermediate hosts. *Treatment*: Dosing, under proper conditions, with arecoline hydrobromide.

(2) One unarmed tapeworm infests dogs in the Great Lakes region; another occurs in cats and sometimes dogs in New York and Louisiana. The parasites require two intermediate hosts, first a small crustacean, second a fish or an amphibian, reptile, or mammal. The symptoms of infestation are usually not marked in the case of dogs, but cats may be severely affected. *Prevention*: Keep dogs and cats from eating the infected flesh of the second intermediate host. *Treatment*: Dosing, under proper conditions, with oleoresin of male fern.

Roundworms (nematodes)

These are the most injurious parasites of dogs and cats.

(1) Hookworms, of which one is widespread, one occurs in the South, and one in the North, are the most injurious of the roundworms. The eggs of hookworms pass out in the feces of the animal, and the infective larvae are taken up in contaminated feed or water or penetrate the skin. Dogs may be infected even before birth. Marked anemia from the bloodsucking activities of the parasite in the intestines, and from internal hemorrhage, is the principal result. *Prevention*: Sanitation and prompt disposal or feces; sterilization of contaminated soil in runs with strong salt brine. *Treatment*: Dosing, under suitable conditions, with tetrachlorethylene or normal butyl chloride.

(2) Large intestinal roundworms (ascarids): One species infests dogs, one cats, and one both dogs and cats. The eggs pass out with the feces, develop to an infective stage, and are swallowed with contaminated feed or water. The larvae migrate extensively in the body, affecting the liver, lungs, and intestines and causing unthriftiness, intestinal disturbances, obstruction of the intestines, sometimes pneumonia, and other injuries. They are especially injurious to young animals. *Prevention*: Sanitation and prompt disposal of feces. *Treatment*: As for hookworms.

(3) The dog whipworm infests the cecum, or blind gut, and is probably injurious, though the symptoms of infestation are vague. Infection is acquired as in the case of ascarids. *Prevention*: As for ascarids. *Treatment*: Dosing, under suitable conditions, with normal butyl chloride.

(4) The heart worm infests dogs and occasionally cats, usually occurring in the heart and the pulmonary artery. It is most abundant in the South and along the Atlantic coast as far north as New York. Active larvae are discharged directly into the blood stream, from which they are picked up by mosquitoes and possibly by fleas. Symptoms include gasping, coughing, collapse, and nervous disturbances. *Prevention*: Keep dogs free of fleas and confine them at night in mosquito-proof kennels. *Treatment*: Injections of antimony

compounds (dangerous to dogs–should be given only by a veterinarian).

(5) The esophageal worm of dogs, found in tumors in the esophagus and stomach, passes part of its life in the body of a beetle. In dogs it can produce such serious consequences as pleurisy, peritonitis suffocation, rupture of blood vessels.

(6) Lungworms are relatively rare in dogs and cats but may be important in some areas. Coughing, wheezing, general unthriftiness, and emaciation are among the symptoms of infestation.

(7) The kidney worm is not a common parasite of dogs in the United States. It occurs in the abdominal cavity and sometimes the kidney and may cause serious injury.

(8) An eye worm that infests other animals has also been reported in dogs and cats in California. It lives under the eyelid and in the tear ducts, sometimes causing serious injury and blindness.

In general, less is known about the life histories of the esophageal worms, lungworms, kidney worms, and eye worms than about the other worm parasites of dogs and cats, and the authors give no specific recommendations for control or treatment.

The authors describe a new treatment, consisting of hydrogen peroxide administered as an enema, that is reported to be effective for all types of worms that infest the intestinal tract. It should be used with caution.

Mange of Dogs

Dogs are attacked by three kinds of mites, each of which causes a different kind of mange, described by Price and Bishopp.

(1) Sarcoptic mange, or scabies, caused by a tiny mite the female of which burrows into the skin, is characterized at first by red points, then by small blisters, and finally by scabs and crusts, baldness, and a peculiar odour. Itching is intense, the whole body may eventually be involved, body functions are upset, and the disease may be fatal if untreated. It can also be transmitted to human beings.

(2) Ear mange is caused by a larger mite that lives deep in the ear canal, where it punctures the skin. Bacterial invasions

may follow, producing inflammation of the inner ear and even of the brain.

(3) Demodectic or red mange, the most common of the three, is caused by a wormlike mite that lives in the hair follicles and sebaceous glands. The disease is characterized by gradually spreading bald patches, a coppery colour of the skin, pustules (pimples), and invasions by pus-forming bacteria, which produce poisons that may eventually cause death.

Mange of dogs should be diagnosed and treated by a veterinarian. Ear mange is the easiest to cure, and various remedies containing phenol, carbon tetrachloride, or rotenone are used. Sulfur in various forms or rotenone in ointments or washes is used for sarcoptic mange. Red mange is the hardest to cure; rotenone used in various ways is a promising remedy, and a combination of carbolic acid, sulfur, oil of tar, kerosene, and linseed oil is sometimes employed. A good diet, comfortable quarters, and adequate disinfection of the premises should accompany any treatment for mange.

Ticks Affecting Dogs

Bishopp and Smith describe eight different species of ticks that attack dogs, but most people know them all as "dog ticks" or "wood ticks." Practically all of them also bite human beings. Several carry Rocky Mountain spotted fever and tularemia, or rabbit fever. All have somewhat similar habits and life histories and must feed on blood to reproduce.

The American dog tick, the most widely distributed and abundant, is found particularly along the Atlantic and Gulf coasts, in the Mississippi Valley, and along the Pacific coast south of Oregon. It carries Rocky Mountain spotted fever and tularemia, though these diseases do not occur everywhere and only one tick in several hundred is actually infected. An engorged female deposits 3,000 to 6,000 eggs in a mass on the ground, and the seed ticks and nymphs feed on meadow mice and other rodents. The adults feed on dogs, other large animals, and human beings. Larvae and nymphs can live a year without feeding and adults over 2 years.

The best way to control these and other ticks is to immerse or wash the dog regularly twice a week in a derris dip (1 ounce of mild soap and 2 ounces of derris or cube powder to each gallon of warm water). The liquid will keep for 2 or 3 weeks in a tank in a dark place, but if no dipping tank is available the dog can be washed thoroughly in a tub. The authors describe the procedure in detail. In lieu of a dip, derris, or cube powder may be applied as a dust. Ticks can also be removed individually with tweezers and dropped in turpentine or kerosene, care being taken to prevent infection. Destruction of rodents, keeping vegetation closely cut or grazed, burning over, and spraying vegetation with nicotine sulfate are all useful control measures under certain circumstances.

Other ticks described are the Rocky Mountain spotted fever tick (Rocky Mountain region), the Pacific coast tick (California and southern Oregon), the black-legged tick (Eastern and Southern States), the California black-legged tick (Pacific coast), the Gulf coast tick (Gulf and southern Atlantic coasts), and the lone star tick (Eastern States as far west as Texas). For each of these, certain of the control measures recommended for the American dog tick are applicable.

Two other ticks require different treatment. The spinose ear tick, which gets deep into the dog's ear, can be killed with a few drops of derris or cube powder mixed in medicinal mineral oil and dropped into the ear; or a mixture of pine tar and cottonseed oils may be used. The brown dog tick, which occurs all over the United States, can live entirely indoors in heated buildings, needs no other animal except the dog on which to complete its life cycle, and is especially difficult to eradicate. The derris dip should be used at 3-day intervals. Wooden kennels should be sprayed with undiluted creosote oil and metal kennels with triple-strength creosote dip (or a blowtorch may be used along cracks). In dwelling houses, pyrethrum-kerosene sprays and powder may be employed to combat infestations.

Fleas

Human fleas, dog fleas, cat fleas, and the sticktight fleas of poultry all attack dogs and cats, and the human flea can also breed on hogs. The cat flea, dog flea, and human flea serve as intermediate hosts for the dog tapeworm, which can infect human beings. All three of these flea species can–although they usually do not–carry bubonic plague. Fleas are also apparently associated with summer eczema of dogs. To this list of evils must be added the torment caused by fleas and the fact that, uncontrolled, they can completely overrun houses and farm buildings. Why put up with them, asks Bishopp, when they can easily be suppressed?

For dogs and cats, scatter a small amount of derris, cube, or fresh pyrethrum powder next to the skin along the neck and back; or wash the animal in water containing derris or cube powder and soap. Repeat the treatment every 10 days or 2 weeks. For hogs, sprinkle the back lightly with crude petroleum or strained crankcase oil. For poultry, destroy the fleas on the premises.

Flea eggs are deposited on the host but soon drop off and hatch out tiny maggotlike larvae, which become pupae about the size of a wheat kernel and finally adult fleas. To kill fleas and larvae on the premises, use a creosote oil spray. In infested buildings, such as homes, where creosote oil would be damaging, scatter flaked naphthalene liberally–about 5 pounds to a room–and close up and vacate the building for at least 48 hours. Close cutting of grass will usually kill fleas in lawns, or the grass can be sprayed with nicotine sulfate.

Running Fits (Fright Disease)

The symptoms of running fits, also known as fright disease, barking fits, furious fits, and canine hysteria, are rather accurately indicated by the names given to this nervous disease; for no apparent reason the dog suddenly starts running and barking, then hides in a dark place, or may have spasms and convulsions. Attacks recur and the condition may last for years. Many persons have mistakenly confused it with rabies. No cause is definitely known, though the disease has been attributed to infection, heredity, inbreeding, circulatory disturbances, deficiency of vitamin A or vitamin B_1, indigestion, intestinal poisoning, parasites, estrum, and various irritations and excitements.

Among measures for treatment and prevention suggested by Stein are a good diet, high in fresh meat, milk, and eggs; good regulation of the bowels; correction of any parasitic infestation; occasional use of small amounts of cod-liver oil, calcium lactate, and yeast for dogs that are kept confined. During an attack the dog should be left unmolested in a dark room, and afterwords it should be kept as quiet as possible. If treatment, such as intestinal irrigation or the administration of nerve sedatives, is necessary, it should be undertaken only by a veterinarian.

Non-Parasitic Skin Diseases of Dogs and Cats

When a dog or a cat develops some skin disease, most people are inclined to call it either mange or eczema. As a matter of fact, it might be any one of a number of other skin maladies, some of which are common, others uncommon; and expert diagnosis, including a microscopic examination or even a culture test, may be necessary to determine the exact trouble, and hence the treatment. Moreover, of the 11 non-parasitic diseases discussed by Stein in this article, only 2, ringworm and favus, have absolutely specific causes–in these two cases, fungi. The other nine conditions– alopecia (falling hair), dandruff, dermatitis (inflammation of the skin), eczema, impetigo, seborrhea, acne, lip ulceration of cats, and urticaria (hives)–may all be due to various causes. In other words, the name of the disease does not identify any particular cause, but simply designates a group of symptoms.

These symptoms are described in the article, which discusses the known or possible causes in each case and the treatments that may be used. Prevention, of course, depends on avoiding or eliminating the causes of a given condition.

Nutritional Diseases of Dogs and Cats

Much more is known about the nutrition of dogs, Earle points out, than about that of cats, but it is assumed that both suffer from the same nutritional diseases. In practice, such diseases are usually due to two or more deficiencies occurring at the same time rather than to one, as in the laboratory. A well-balanced diet of natural foodstuffs is the best preventive and the best cure, though it may be advisable to use pure vitamins for emergency treatment. The author gives the quantitative vitamin requirements wherever possible and suggests common food sources from which the vitamins and minerals are obtained. The following nutritional diseases are discussed in some detail:

Rickets in young dogs and cats, as in other animals and human beings, is due to a deficiency of calcium, phosphorus, or vitamin D, or to an unbalance between the two minerals. The condition can be detected much earlier by X-ray than by clinical symptoms.

Eclampsia, a malady of female dogs and cats at the time of parturition, is apparently due to a deficiency of calcium and a vitamin D disturbance.

Scurvy, or a condition like it, occasionally occurs in dogs and can be relieved by the administration of vitamin C. Dogs are supposed to manufacture their own vitamin C, but there may sometimes be a failure in normal functioning of the animal organism.

Nutritional anemia is commonly associated with a deficiency of iron or copper, or a prolonged shortage of proteins necessary for the formation of red blood cells. The necessary iron can easily be supplied by meat, especially liver. Apparently a deficiency of vitamin B_6 can cause a certain type of anemia, associated with blacktongue.

Vitamin A deficiency is often not diagnosed until it is so advanced that the animal may fail to recover even under treatment; xerophthalmia, a serious eye disease, is an advanced symptom. Conditions due to a partial deficiency are particularly hard to diagnose. Not much work has been done with night blindness in dogs, but Earle suggests that it might be studied as an early symptom of a deficiency of this vitamin.

Thiamin (B_1) deficiency produces a disease in dogs that closely parallels beri-beri in human beings. Marked loss of appetite is an early symptom of a deficiency of this vitamin in dogs; others include nervousness and fatigue. There is some evidence that thiamin deficiency may be a factor in fright disease.

Riboflavin (B_2) deficiency results in a redness and dry scaliness of the skin, with severe symptoms such as a staggering gait and collapse in acute stages.

Blacktongue, a disease that apparently parallels pellagra in human beings, can be cured and prevented by a diet containing adequate amounts of nicotinic acid and other B vitamins.

Other vitamin B deficiencies. For normal health, dogs require pantothenic acid and biotin (the so-called anti-gray-hair factor) as well as the other B vitamins mentioned.

Chapter 1

RABIES AND ITS CONTROL

H.W. Schoening [1]

[1] *H.W. Schoening is Chief, Pathological Division, Bureau of Animal Industry.*

Rabies is an outstanding example of a dangerous disease which could be controlled or eventually eradicated in this country but which is not under control because of failure to impose and thoroughly carry out uniform regulations. Here is an account of the disease and the control measures it demands.

Through its veterinary services, Federal, State, and private, the United States has been outstanding among the countries of the world in controlling and eradicating animal diseases and, generally speaking, has attained a freedom from infectious animal diseases second to none. There is one animal disease that is far too prevalent in this country, however, and that disease is rabies. The irony of the situation lies in the fact that rabies is controllable and even eradicable if present knowledge were applied. Outstanding livestock sanitarians and scientists visiting this country from abroad have from time to time expressed amazement at the prevalence of rabies in the United States–a country in which such great strides have been made in the control or eradication of foot-and-mouth disease, tuberculosis, brucellosis, and other contagious diseases of animals.

Before entering into a discussion of the reasons for the prevalence of rabies in this country it would be well to discuss the known facts concerning the disease and methods for its control.

Nature and Characteristics of Rabies

Rabies or hydrophobia is ages old; it was described several centuries before the beginning of the Christian era as a dread disease. Only in modern times, however, through the brilliant work of Pasteur and others following him, has exact information become available on the cause, transmission, and control of rabies.

The disease is primarily one of the dog, although a wide variety of species are susceptible to infection, including man. Rabies has been reported in the cat, cow, horse, mule, sheep, goat, hog, wolf, fox, coyote, hyena, skunk, monkey, deer, antelope, camel, bear, elk, polecat, bat, squirrel, hare, rabbit, rat, mouse, jackal, badger, marmot, wood-chuck, porcupine, weasel, hedgehog, gopher, raccoon, owl, hawk, chicken, pigeon, and stork. It is definitely recognized, however, that the chief disseminator of rabies is the dog and that when rabies is once controlled in this species it will cease to be of any great importance from an economic or public health standpoint. It should be recognized, however, that once the disease becomes established in a wild species, a serious situation develops, and strenuous efforts must be made to control it in the species affected.

The disease is caused by a filtrable virus–a type of infective agent sometimes called an ultramicroscopic virus, capable of passing through certain filters that retain ordinary bacteria and not rendered visible by any of our present-day microscopes. The infective agent is found in the saliva of affected animals, and under natural conditions, as it exists in dogs, the disease is produced by the bite of a rabid animal or by contact with the saliva of a rabid animal. The bite makes a wound in which the virus in the saliva is deposited.

The period of incubation, that is, the time between exposure to infection and the first appearance of symptoms of the disease, is variable. It may be as short as 2 weeks or as long as many months. The majority of cases, however, develop within a 3-month period.

Every animal or person bitten does not necessarily develop the disease, and the percentage of fatalities has been variously estimated. According to Hogyes, the proportion of persons who contract the disease after being bitten by rabid dogs and not treated is conservatively estimated at 15 percent. The percentage is considerably higher in man following bites by the wolf. From 35 to 45 per cent of the dogs, 40 per cent of the horses, 36 per cent of the hogs, and 25 to 30 per cent of the cattle bitten by rabid animals contract the disease, making a general average of about 35 per cent for these animals. Whether an individual animal contracts the disease depends in part on the location and size of the wound, the amount of hemorrhage produced, and various other conditions. In general, the nearer the bite to the central nervous system and the deeper the wound, the greater is the danger of infection. In cases in which the hemorrhage resulting from the bite is profuse, there is a possibility that the virus will be washed out of the wound. Also, exact information is not available on whether the virus of rabies is constantly present in the saliva of a rabid animal. It may be variable in both quantity and virulence.

After being deposited in the wound, the virus remains latent for an extremely variable period of time, which depends on the size and depth of the wound as well as its location and the amount of virulent saliva introduced. Experiments have proved that the virus follows the course of the nerves to the spinal cord and along the latter to the brain before the symptoms appear. Gerlach, who collected statistics from a large number of cases, found the period between the bite and the appearance of the first symptom to vary from 14 to 285 days.

Rabies in Dogs

Symptoms

In dogs the first symptom of rabies may be a change in behaviour. The animal may become restless, somewhat nervous, and excitable. This condition may subside, to reappear within a short time. The dog's disposition may change; a friendly dog may become irritable and snappy, whereas an ordinarily less amiable animal may become friendly. Later the animal may have a tendency to wander, and may disappear for a day or two, returning exhausted and considerably emaciated. The dog may seek dark corners and hide. At times a characteristic change in the bark, or "change in voice," is noted, which might best be described as a different tone.

Later the animal develops partial paralysis, staggers, and has difficulty in drinking, although it may make efforts to lap water. It staggers around until complete paralysis sets in and the symptoms finally terminate in death. Since the virus attacks the brain and spinal cord and sets up degenerative changes, the various symptoms noted-excitability, convulsions, and paralysis-can be correlated with changes in the central nervous system. The inability to swallow results from paralysis of the muscles of the throat.

Although the term "hydrophobia" means fear of water, its application to the disease in dogs appears to be a misnomer, since affected dogs show no fear of water. The use of the term probably has its origin in the fact that dogs and human beings affected with the disease have been observed to develop convulsions through their unsuccessful efforts to drink. Even the mere thought of drinking on the part of human beings has been responsible for convulsions, and a dread of water or drinking becomes established in many patients.

In the furious form of the disease, the animal is aggressive, will snap at various objects that are placed before it, and will attack dogs, people, or any object. When confined in a cage, it may attack the bars with such vigour that it may break some of its teeth.

In this form of the disease, the dog's tendency to roam, its restlessness, and its inclination to bite, particularly anything moving, lead to the dissemination of the disease over a wide area. It should be remembered that rabies may manifest itself in a number of forms and that the symptoms described are those of a typical case. Many animals affected with rabies do not exhibit these symptoms. The symptoms may be more or less masked and perhaps be manifested eventually only by paralysis.

In the dumb form of rabies, paralytic symptoms are the outstanding feature. The dog is not vicious, has no tendency to bite or roam, and is not excitable; in fact, it may be the opposite. The outstanding clinical feature of so-called dumb rabies is paralysis of the lower jaw, or "dropped jaw." The animal's mouth stays open from about an inch to 3 or 4 inches. It can be closed with the hands, but the dog has lost the power to close its own jaw. Many times this is mistakenly thought to be due to a bone in the throat, and many persons have exposed themselves to the virus of rabies by examining the mouth and throat for the presence of a bone. Usually a dog with a bone stuck in its mouth or throat will continually make efforts with its paws or otherwise to remove the object, whereas in dumb rabies the animal makes no motion about the head with its paws. An animal with a dropped jaw should be viewed with suspicion, and no examination should be made of the throat; such an animal should be taken immediately to a veterinarian for a diagnosis.

In addition to the dropped jaw, in the dumb form of rabies the animal shows evidence of paralysis of the hindquarters and forequarters within a few days. It eventually becomes completely paralyzed and dies.

The course of the disease in both the furious and the dumb forms is usually short, the animal dying within 3 to 7 days.

Transmission

As already noted, the virus of rabies is found in the saliva of the rabid dog. The presence, quantity, and virulence of the virus in the saliva may vary considerably in different animals and even in the same animal during the course of the disease. After death the virus is found in the brain and spinal cord. Evidence has been presented to show that the virus of rabies may be present in the animal some days before clinical symptoms are apparent. It has been demonstrated that the bite of a dog may be infectious at least 3 days before the dog manifests symptoms of rabies, and in one case in the Pasteur Institute at Athens, Greece, infection was found to be present in the saliva 8 days before the dog showed signs of the disease. Exact information is not available on the regularity with which the virus appears in the saliva before animals show evidence of the disease, nor is there exact information on the persistence of the virus in the saliva of animals showing clinical symptoms.

For a dog to transmit rabies through a bite, it must itself be affected with the disease. Bites of dogs not affected with rabies cannot result in the transmission of rabies. The bite of a normal dog can be disregarded from the standpoint of the possibility of its producing rabies and need only be treated as any other injury would be.

Diagnosis

It is of great importance to establish definitely the presence or absence of rabies infection in dogs that have bitten people, so that proper measures can be taken. Since the diagnosis of the disease can be based on both clinical and laboratory examinations, it is essential that the dog be kept under observation by a qualified veterinarian. Since rabies is a fatal disease and an affected animal will shortly die, the brain can then be subjected to laboratory examination for the presence of special changes, which are indicated by the presence of Negri bodies in certain portions. This valuable laboratory diagnostic procedure was developed through the work of an Italian scientist named Negri, who first called attention to the presence of these bodies in the brain of rabid dogs. Although the bodies are specific in the diagnosis of rabies, they may in certain cases be few in number, particularly if the animals have been destroyed in the early stages of the disease. For this reason it is advisable to allow the disease to progress to its termination or to a well-advanced stage so that the laboratory diagnosis can be conclusive.

Since it has been reported that the virus of rabies may be in the saliva of a rabid dog 8 days before the animal shows any clinical evidence of the disease, it is important that dogs suspected of having rabies or dogs that have bitten people be held in strict quarantine in suitable strong, tight quarters for a period of 2 weeks in order that a correct diagnosis may be made. It is essential that the quarters in which the animal is confined be well-made and escape-proof, since animals developing rabies will make extraordinary efforts to gain their freedom. If a rabid dog is not properly housed, it may work its way out and disappear, to die some days later at a distant point without ever being identified; and this would make the handling of a case of a person bitten by the dog more difficult. The fact that the dog had escaped would in itself be some indication that it might have been rabid, but in the absence of proof, an uncertain situation develops.

Rabies in Cattle

Both furious and dumb rabies are met with in cattle, the former being the more common. A sharp distinction cannot always be drawn between the two, however, as the furious type usually merges into the dumb owing to the paralysis that always appears before death. The typical cases of dumb rabies are those in which the paralysis occurs at the beginning of the attack and remains until the death of the animal. The disease first manifests itself by loss of appetite, stopping of the secretion of milk, great restlessness, anxiety, manifestations of fear, and a change in disposition. This preliminary stage is followed in a day or two by the stage of excitation or madness, which is indicated by increasing restlessness, loud bellowing with a peculiar change in the sound of the voice, violent butting with the head and pawing the ground, and an insane tendency to attack other animals, although the desire to bite is not so marked in cattle as in dogs. About the fourth day the animal usually becomes quieter, and the walk is stiff, unsteady, and swaying, showing that the final paralysis is coming on. Loss of flesh is very rapid, and even during the short course of the disease the animal becomes extremely emaciated. The temperature is never elevated but usually remains about normal or even subnormal. Finally, there is complete paralysis of the hindquarters, the animal is unable to rise and, except for irregular convulsive movements, lies in a comatose condition, and dies usually in 4 to 6 days after the appearance of the first symptoms.

Rabies in Cats

When the disease attacks cats, they generally hide under the furniture or in some dark corner, and there they may die unobserved in a day or two. As a rule, however, the disease in cats implies danger for human beings. The rabid cat becomes very bellicose; from the dark corner where it has hidden it will suddenly attack animals or persons, especially children, jumping up to the face and inflicting severe wounds with its teeth and claws. In the violence of this attack it frequently bites itself. The rabid cat nearly loses its voice, being able only to mew hoarsely. Later it loses its appetite, has difficulty in swallowing, becomes emaciated, and succumbs within several days with symptoms of paralysis.

Rabies in Wildlife

As has been previously stated, rabies may appear in wildlife, since a wide variety of wild animals, already listed, are susceptible. In certain parts of the country the appearance of the disease among wildlife has caused considerable loss of livestock, as well as presenting a human health hazard.

In 1915, according to the United States Biological Survey, epizootics, or severe outbreaks, among wild animals, especially coyotes, appeared in Oregon, California, Nevada, and Idaho. In one feed lot alone, a single rabid coyote bit and caused the loss of 27 steers. There were further outbreaks in 1921 to 1928, and more or less serious outbreaks have been reported since that time. Outbreaks of rabies in foxes occurred in Maine in 1934 and in Massachusetts in 1935.

More recently, in 1940, a serious outbreak of rabies among foxes occurred in several of the Southern States, the worst center of infection being in Georgia, although adjoining areas in South Carolina and Alabama reported infection in foxes. Just where the infection originated is not known, but of 291 fox heads examined in Georgia up to December 1940, 88, or 30.2 percent, were found to be affected with rabies. At least 90 head of livestock were reported to have developed the disease from exposure to rabid foxes, and it is probable that the total far exceeds that number. In addition, the Georgia Department of Public Health furnished antirabic treatment to 17 persons bitten by or exposed to rabid foxes.

The problem of the control of rabies in wildlife has aspects different from those in the control of rabies in dogs. As the first step, it is necessary to reduce the number of wild animals in the area, particularly the affected species, by trapping, poisoning, and other means. Effective cooperation between Federal, State, and local agencies and the public at large is an essential feature of control of the disease.

Post Mortem Appearance

In rabies no constant or definite lesions are observed on post mortem examination. In fact the alterations are slight, variable, and almost absent at times, so that, unless there is a definite history of characteristic symptoms, a positive diagnosis cannot be made without recourse to microscopic examination or animal inoculations with material from the brain of the suspected animal. The most suggestive indication of rabies is the presence in the stomach of unusual bodies, such as stones, wood, earth, cloth, iron, and feathers. Frequently the stomach is empty of food but distended with material of this character. Its mucous membrane is frequently inflamed, and at times a marked reddening of the folds of the stomach, with or without erosions, is noticed. There may also be an inflammation of the covering of the brain and spinal cord as well as of the mucous lining of the mouth, throat, and respiratory tract. The feet of rabid dogs may present sores and bruises, denoting extensive travel during the period of roving. The heart and the surrounding membrane (pericardium) are often inflamed, but these and similar lesions are more frequently due to the condition of the animal before dying than to any specific alteration. The carcass undergoes rapid decomposition.

Transmission by Milk and Meat

From the reports in the literature it appears that in a few instances rabies virus has been found in the milk or udder tissue of lactating animals. This subject has been investigated by a number of workers in different parts of the world at various times. The great majority have failed to find the virus of rabies in the milk or in udder tissue. In 1934 the Bureau of Animal Industry conducted some experimental work on this point, since it is important to know whether milk can carry the infection.

The virus of rabies was inoculated into the tongues of two milking cows on different occasions. Samples of milk were taken from these animals during the course of the disease at frequent intervals. In addition, milk from the cistern and udder tissues of the animals was collected at death, and samples were inoculated into the brains of rabbits. All these inoculations resulted negatively. A calf and four pigs were fed the milk taken daily from the two cows from the time of exposure to the virus to the time of death from rabies. The mucous membrane of the mouth of two of the pigs and the calf was scarified frequently, producing minute wounds in the mouth parts, but in no case did these animals show any harmful effects from the consumption of this milk. In further tests, rabies virus in the form of a brain emulsion was added to milk and then fed to 4 hogs. Abrasions were produced mechanically on the mucous surfaces of the mouths of these animals. In no case did the animals show any evidence of rabies. It appears, therefore, from the information available, that although the virus of rabies may at times be found in milk, the chances of such a happening are remote, and from a practical standpoint there would appear to be little danger in the consumption of milk from even a rabid animal. Milk secretion is usually considerably diminished at the clinical appearance of the disease, with the result that in most cases none of the animal's milk has been consumed after symptoms have appeared. However, the milk from a rabid or suspected cow naturally should be condemned as unfit for consumption.

The same position should be taken with regard to the meat or meat food products of a rabid or suspected animal. The disposition of farm animals that have been exposed to the bites of a rabid dog but do not show signs of the disease also presents a practical sanitary police problem. The International Rabies Conference held in Paris in 1927 under the auspices of the Health Committee of the League of Nations made the following recommendation on this point: "Animals bitten by rabid animals, whether, treated or not after the bite, should not be butchered between the eighth day and, at the very least, the end of the third month following the bite."[2] Since this may be a problem of considerable importance in areas where rabies exists, the recommendations quoted form a basis for methods of procedure.

Prevalence of Rabies in the United States

Exact information on the prevalence of rabies in the United States is difficult to obtain. The Bureau of Animal Industry collected the available information on the incidence of rabies in the various States in 1938 and 1939 through a questionnaire submitted to the various State livestock sanitary officials and State health officers. It is very probable that there were more cases of the disease in the United States than were reported by the officials with whom contacts were made. Table 1 gives the number of cases of rabies by States in the various species in the calendar years 1938 and 1939.

Rabies in Other Countries

After the first World War rabies became widespread, chiefly in central Europe. Owing to strict sanitary regulations, the incidence of the disease has been greatly reduced. Northern countries, including Great Britain, Denmark, Sweden, and Norway, have been free from rabies for the last decade. The disease has not appeared recently in the Netherlands, Belgium, and Switzerland, but it is still present to a limited extent in Germany and Austria. In the southern and eastern countries of Europe it is of frequent occurrence, although its incidence has been reduced under that following the last war. In certain South American countries the disease is seen in cattle and horses as a result of infection by the vampire bat. Rabies is reported in Asia, Japan, and parts of Africa, but Australia has remained free from it.

Control Measures

The control of rabies in the United States at the present time lies within the authority of the States. In many instances this authority is divided between the State livestock sanitary service and the State department of health. The laws and regulations governing the control

---

2 RESOLUTIONS ADOPTED BY THE CONFERENCE. League of Nations Health Organ., Internatl. Rabies Conf. Rpts., pp. 7-11. 1927.

Table 1: Cases of rabies reported in the United States, by States, during 1938 and 1939.

State and Year	Dogs Number	Cattle Number	Horses Number	Sheep Number	Swine Number	Cats Number	Goats Number	Miscellaneous[1] Number	Man Number	Total Number
Alabama										
1938	(2)	(2)	(2)	(2)	(2)	(2)	(2)	(2)	2	2
1939	,221	5	0	0	0	15	0	0	3	244
Arizona										
1938	(3)	(3)	(3)	(3)	(3)	(3)	(3)	(3)	(3)	(3)
1939	9	0	0	0	0	0	0	0	0	9
Arkansas										
1938	256	40	3	80	0	0	0	0	2	381
1939	233	11	2	1	0	9	0	0	0	256
California										
1938	1,576	50	3	56	4	30	6	6	4	1,735
1939	828	17	1	1	2	38	2	10	1	900
Colorado										
1938	2	0	0	0	0	0	0	0	0	2
1939	2	0	0	0	0	0	0	0	0	2
Connecticut										
1938	40	0	0	0	0	2	0	0	0	42
1939	11	0	0	0	0	1	0	0	0	12
Delaware										
1938	3	0	0	0	0	0	0	0	0	3
1939	12	0	1	0	0	0	0	0	0	13

Contd...

Table 1–Contd...

State and Year	Dogs	Cattle	Horses	Sheep	Swine	Cats	Goats	Miscellaneous[1]	Man	Total
	Number	Number	Number	Number	Number	Number	Number	Number	Number	Number
District of Columbia										
1938	2	0	0	0	0	0	0	0	0	2
1939	0	0	0	0	0	0	0	0	0	0
Florida										
1938	311	11	0	0	0	11	0	0	3	336
1939	14	0	0	0	0	3	0	0	0	17
Georgia										
1938	543	13	3	0	2	41	1	1	2	606
1939	434	19	0	0	1	23	0	2	1	482
Idaho										
1938	0	0	0	0	0	0	0	0	0	0
1939	3	0	0	0	0	0	0	0	0	3
Illinois										
1938	645	37	1	0	2	0	0	0	5	690
1939	266	0	0	0	0	0	0	54	2	322
Indiana										
1938	505	63	3	6	16	21	0	2	0	616
1939	329	39	1	3	13	22	2	11	2	422
Iowa										
1938	8	3	1	0	0	1	0	5	0	18
1939	11	8	7	0	4	4	0	15	0	49

Contd...

Table 1–Contd...

State and Year	*Dogs*	*Cattle*	*Horses*	*Sheep*	*Swine*	*Cats*	*Goats*	*Miscellaneous*[1]	*Man*	*Total*
	Number	*Number*	*Number*	*Number*	*Number*	*Number*	*Number*	*Number*	*Number*	*Number*
Kansas										
1938	52	3	0	0	0	1	0	2	0	58
1939	31	7	0	0	0	7	0	6	0	51
Kentucky										
1938	63	4	1	0	4	4	0	5	0	81
1939	73	1	0	1	0	3	0	0	1	79
Louisiana										
1938	130	16	0	0	0	18	0	0	0	164
1939	185	18	2	0	0	7	0	35	2	249
Maine										
1938	1	0	0	0	0	0	0	0	0	1
1939	1	0	0	0	0	0	0	0	0	1
Maryland										
1938	15	2	1	0	0	0	0	0	0	18
1939	1	0	0	0	0	0	0	0	0	1
Massachusetts										
1938	59	1	0	0	0	0	0	0	0	60
1939	39	0	0	0	0	1	0	0	0	40
Michigan										
1938	317	37	6	21	3	4	0	1	4	393
1939	548	43	5	4	7	11	0	0	5	623

Contd...

Table 1–Contd...

State and Year	Dogs	Cattle	Horses	Sheep	Swine	Cats	Goats	Miscellaneous[1]	Man	Total
	Number	Number	Number	Number	Number	Number	Number	Number	Number	Number
Minnesota										
1938	137	4	1	0	5	1	0	0	0	148
1939	16	6	1	0	4	3	1	0	0	31
Mississippi										
1938	250	(4)	(4)	(4)	(4)	(4)	(4)	(4)	3	253
1939	131	12	2	1	0	10	0	0	0	156
Missouri										
1938	(5)	(5)	(5)	(5)	(5)	(5)	(5)	(5)	(5)	0
1939	47	0	0	0	0	0	0	0	0	47
Montana										
1938	0	0	0	0	0	0	0	0	0	0
1939	0	0	0	0	0	0	0	0	0	0
Nebraska										
1938	0	0	0	0	0	0	0	0	0	0
1939	0	0	0	0	0	0	0	0	0	0
Nevada										
1938	0	0	0	0	0	0	0	0	0	0
1939	0	0	0	0	0	0	0	0	0	0
New Hampshire										
1938	6	0	0	0	0	0	0	0	0	6
1939	0	0	0	0	0	0	0	0	0	0

Contd...

Table 1–Contd...

State and Year	Dogs Number	Cattle Number	Horses Number	Sheep Number	Swine Number	Cats Number	Goats Number	Miscellaneous[1] Number	Man Number	Total Number
New Jersey										
1938	563	3	0	0	0	5	2	0	2	575
1939	679	11	0	0	0	0	0	0	2	692
New Mexico										
1938	100	2	0	0	0	0	1	0	0	103
1939	87	3	0	0	0	1	1	0	0	92
New York State										
1938	75	0	0	0	0	0	0	0	0	75
1939	153	1	0	0	0	0	0	0	0	154
New York City										
1938	86	0	0	0	0	3	0	0	1	90
1939	58	0	0	0	0	0	0	0	0	58
North Carolina										
1938	253	12	2	0	0	0	0	0	1	268
1939	235	9	0	0	0	8	1	10	1	264
North Dakota										
1938	1	0	0	0	0	0	0	0	0	1
1939	0	0	0	0	0	0	0	0	0	0
Ohio										
1938	(5)	(5)	(5)	(5)	(5)	(5)	(5)	(5)	3	3
1939	271	15	1	2	0	8	0	8	0	305

Contd...

Table 1–Contd...

State and Year	Dogs Number	Cattle Number	Horses Number	Sheep Number	Swine Number	Cats Number	Goats Number	Miscellaneous[1] Number	Man Number	Total Number
Oklahoma										
1938	233	(4)	(4)	(4)	(4)	(4)	(4)	(4)	1	234
1939	168	21	1	1	3	15	1	6	1	217
Oregon										
1938	9	10	0	0	0	0	0	0	0	19
1939	29	9	0	0	0	1	1	0	0	40
Pennsylvania										
1938	493	3	0	0	1	9	0	0	4	510
1939	420	4	4	0	0	5	0	0	2	435
Rhode Island										
1938	33	0	0	0	0	0	0	0	0	33
1939	17	2	1	0	0	1	0	0	0	21
South Carolina										
1938	348	0	0	0	0	0	0	0	2	350
1939	295	3	0	0	1	10	0	4	4	317
South Dakota										
1938	1	0	0	0	0	0	0	0	0	1
1939	0	0	0	0	0	0	0	0	0	0
Tennessee										
1938	182	15	0	0	0	12	0	0	4	213
1939	237	9	0	2	1	11	0	4	2	266

Contd...

Table 1–Contd...

State and Year	Dogs Number	Cattle Number	Horses Number	Sheep Number	Swine Number	Cats Number	Goats Number	Miscellaneous[1] Number	Man Number	Total Number
Texas										
1938	484	46	5	0	1	32	1	0	0	569
1939	782	55	4	0	0	38	0	4	0	883
Utah										
1938	0	0	0	0	0	0	0	0	0	0
1939	0	0	0	0	0	0	0	0	0	0
Vermont										
1938	0	0	0	0	0	0	0	0	0	0
1939	3	2	0	0	0	0	0	0	0	5
Virginia										
1938	68	(4)	(4)	(4)	(4)	(4)	(4)	(4)	(4)	68
1939	40	3	1	0	0	0	0	0	0	44
Washington										
1938	355	13	0	0	2	4	0	0	1	375
1939	310	17	0	1	2	5	1	0	1	337
West Virginia										
1938	231	7	0	1	1	7	0	0	2	249
1939	130	4	0	0	0	5	0	0	0	139

Contd...

Table 1–Contd...

State and Year	Dogs	Cattle	Horses	Sheep	Swine	Cats	Goats	Miscellaneous[1]	Man	Total
	Number	Number	Number	Number	Number	Number	Number	Number	Number	Number
Wisconsin										
1938	16	18	2	0	1	1	0	22	0	60
1939	24	4	0	0	0	2	0	3	0	33
Wyoming										
1938	0	0	0	0	0	0	0	0	0	0
1939	3	0	0	0	0	0	0	0	0	3
Totals										
1938	8,452	413	32	164	42	207	11	44	47	9,412
1939	7,386	358	[6]36	17	38	269	10	172	30	8,314

[1] Includes coyote, deer, bobcat, fox, squirrel, skunk, wolf, burro, gopher, raccoon, monkey, and civet cat.

[2] No report received on rabies in animals.

[3] Present, but reliable statement cannot be made.

[4] Not separated as to type.

[5] Present, but no statistics available.

[6] Includes 4 mules.

of rabies in the various States are reasonably satisfactory and are based on modern knowledge of the disease. The subject is well covered in the report of the Committee on Rabies of the United States Live Stock Sanitary Association for 1939,[3] from which the following is taken.

No matter how thorough the regulations are which are promulgated for the control of the disease, the regulations in themselves will be of no avail unless the proper machinery is set up for their enforcement. This, the committee believes, is the weak link, generally speaking, in the present method of control of rabies in this country.

The recognized measures for the control of rabies in dogs include:

1. The proper disposition of rabid and suspected rabid dogs and the definite diagnosis of the disease in these animals.
2. The destruction of the definitely known bitten dogs and the strict quarantining or destruction of contact dogs for at least a 6-month period.
3. Strict licensing of all dogs.
4. The impounding and disposal of stray dogs.
5. Strict general quarantine measures over a sufficiently wide area.
6. Muzzling of all dogs in certain areas.
7. To these may be added the use of rabies vaccines.

Not any one of these measures can accomplish the desired end. Except for item 7, the use of rabies vaccines, all the measures must be used in combination. Their successful use will depend on how thoroughly they are applied.

The officials in this country charged with the control of livestock diseases have been successful in eradicating one of the most contagious diseases known, namely, foot-and-mouth disease. This disease has appeared in this country on a number of occasions, involving at times considerable territory, but has always been

[3] UNITED STATES LIVE STOCK SANITARY ASSOCIATION. REPORT OF THE COMMITTEE ON RABIES. 43d Ann. Meeting U.S. Live Stock Sanit. Assoc. Proc., pp. 151-161. 1939.

successfully eradicated. The methods used in the eradication of this disease, if applied to rabies, would result in the control and possibly the eventual eradication of the disease. It is felt that the incidence of the disease at least would be reduced to such a point that it would no longer be an economic or public health problem.

In order to follow out such measures in the control of rabies, it is essential that sufficient machinery and funds be available. It is not the purpose of this committee at this time to make any recommendations as to what this machinery should be but it is merely intended to bring out the points necessary to accomplish the desired end. After reviewing the questionnaires from the various States, the committee believes that there are not at the present time, in any State where rabies exists to any appreciable extent, sufficient funds and machinery to carry out a proper control programme.

The Prophylactic Vaccination of Dogs Against Rabies

Prophylactic vaccination of dogs in communities where outbreaks of rabies exist is predicated on the reduction of the susceptibility of dogs in that area to the disease. If rabies vaccines, for example, are only a certain per cent effective, it could be assumed that, depending on the number of dogs vaccinated, the number of susceptible dogs would be decreased by that percent. The fewer the susceptible animals, the fewer the number of animals that would become infected and the less chance the disease has for spreading.

The magnitude of a rabies-control programme in this country is realized by the committee. Rabies has flourished in many parts of the country for years, and we may be faced with factors and problems which have not been apparent in other countries where the disease has appeared only for a short time and then has been eradicated. Rabies vaccines may well play an important role in a well-regulated control programme. As an example of the probable value of the use of vaccines in controlling rabies, a recent article comes to attention from Hungary concerning a report on rabies which has been in evidence in that country for many years in spite of vigorous measures for its control. It has been only in the past few years when compulsory prophylactic vaccination was instituted in certain areas that the disease has been reduced to a minimum. In this case, of course, vaccination was only an added means of control, the other sanitary policy measures being vigorously pursued at the same time.

The committee states emphatically that the use of rabies vaccines alone, no matter how effective, cannot control the disease, but that such vaccines can be used to advantage in some communities and under certain conditions in conjunction with other standard measures. The State-wide compulsory vaccination of dogs is not considered advisable as practiced at the present time. Its compulsory use in restricted communities should be approached with caution and only on a sound basis of administration.

In the report of the same committee for 1940[4] the following information concerning the control of rabies is given:

It is realized that it is not possible at this time and in the present state of rabies control in the various States to prescribe hard and fast regulations, since local conditions, with particular reference to the presence or absence of rabies, may make it advisable to modify certain of the regulations. The following proposed regulations, therefore, should be considered in this light:

1. All dogs shall be licensed annually. The fee shall be at least $1 for a male, $1 for a spayed female, and $2 for an unspayed female.
2. The license tag issued when the dog is licensed must be affixed to the collar of the dog and worn at all times when the animal is on public property.
3. All unlicensed dogs or dogs not wearing license tags shall be either humanely destroyed or impounded and disposed of as follows: Animals shall be kept 48 hours (or 72 or 96 hours) and if not claimed within that time shall be humanely destroyed. If an animal is claimed by its owner and has not been licensed, such a dog may be returned to the owner upon the payment of a license fee and a collection and maintenance charge of $2. A licensed dog claimed shall be returned to the owner upon payment of $1 collection charge. (In this connection it may be advisable to assess a penalty against the owner of the dog for violation of the dog regulations. It is also well to consider the possibility of rabies being spread through the return of impounded dogs to their

[4] UNITED STATES LIVE STOCK SANITARY ASSOCIATION. REPORT OF THE COMMITEE ON RABIES. 44th Ann. Meeting U.S. Live Stock Sanit. Assoc. Proc. pp. 52-58. 1940.

owners and through the practice of selling dogs from the pound. Serious consideration should be given to these points, but they probably can best be handled as local conditions warrant.)

4. A sufficient full-time personnel shall be available to properly control stray dogs and unlicensed dogs as provided above.
5. In the event that rabies is reported or suspected in a dog, it shall be the duty of the official in charge to have definitely determined whether or not the animal is rabid. In the event that rabies is established, a thorough inquiry should be made immediately insofar as possible into the movements of the rabid dog so that all dogs known to have beep bitten by or exposed to the rabid dog may be destroyed or kept in quarantine or otherwise treated as hereinafter provided. A quarantine of at least 60 days shall be placed over an area covering the possible movements of the said rabid dog. This quarantine shall provide that all dogs be kept on the premises of the owner, or, when upon public property, shall be held on a leash not over 6 feet long in the hands of a competent person.

   Dogs not definitely known to have been bitten but which have had contact with a rabid dog may be kept in strict quarantine on the premises of the owner for a period of not less than 6 months. Such an animal in addition may be given a series of vaccination treatments by a qualified veterinarian. In this event the quarantine period may be reduced to 2 months. Dogs may not be removed from the quarantined area without specific permission from the constituted authority.
6. *Funds*: There shall be ample funds available for immediate use at all times for the proper carrying out of these regulations. These funds shall be consistent with the size of the community. In addition to this, there shall be set aside a sum of money for the specific purpose of controlling outbreaks of rabies as they might occur. This money shall be available at all times and shall not be used for any other purpose than controlling such outbreaks. This money might come from regularly appropriated State funds labeled for this specific purpose or from dog-tax revenues or from any

source that seems consistent with procedures in the State. In any event, it shall be available at all times in sufficient amounts to meet any expected need.

7. *Personnel*: Since rabies is an animal disease, the veterinary profession shall be represented in the personnel concerned with the control of the disease. The control of rabies in a State shall be fixed in an authority with power to work in any section of the State and to call for such local cooperation as may be feasible or desirable. In outbreaks in communities, due notice of such outbreak and quarantines that might be imposed shall be given publicity and in all possible ways brought to the attention of the public at large and the dog owner in particular.
8. *Vaccination*: When thought advisable or desirable, prophylactic vaccination of dogs may be encouraged or advocated on a voluntary basis. Vaccinated dogs, however, shall not enjoy any special privileges because of such vaccination, since vaccination is considered to be only an adjunct in any programme for the control of rabies.
9. The authority in the State charged with the control of rabies shall notify the authorities in the several States of outbreaks of rabies and their location as they occur, together with the date or dates the quarantine is lifted. All transportation companies in a State shall be notified of outbreaks of rabies and the quarantine regulations imposed governing such outbreaks.

Vaccination of Dogs Against Rabies

Vaccination against rabies dates back to the work of Pasteur, and the method for persons exposed to the disease (the Pasteur treatment) has been in use many years, but its use is limited to human beings. It consists of a number of daily injections of a specially prepared vaccine. In recent years several modifications of Pasteur's vaccine have been in use, and good results have been reported. These methods have also been applied for years to dogs and other animals following exposure to the disease.

In 1921 the single-injection prophylactic vaccination (the one-shot method) against rabies was described by two Japanese investigators, Umeno and Doi, and was introduced into this country by Eichhorn and Lyon in 1922. This type of vaccination has for its purpose the development of immunity in dogs previous to exposure to rabies infection. Although measures are available for the control of rabies without the use of vaccination, in many communities in the past, owing to lack of funds and of cooperation of dog owners and others, these measures have not been carried out as vigorously as they should have been, and the disease under these conditions has been brought under control only after considerable time. In recent years, in order to improve their methods of control, many authorities have enlisted prophylactic vaccination as an adjunct.

Since its introduction in the United States, the prophylactic vaccination of dogs has had extensive use. The vaccines prepared in this country are killed vaccines, the killing agent being either phenol or chloroform. Considerable experimental work has been done with these vaccines, both in dogs and more recently in other animals in the laboratory. Although there has at times been some disagreement in results, particularly with laboratory animals, the results of tests on dogs indicate that this method of vaccination has definite value. It should be remembered, however, as noted in the committee report, that the immunity produced by vaccination in dogs is relative and differs in different dogs. Occasional reactions from the vaccine itself have been observed, chiefly paralysis, which has been for the most part transitory but has caused a few deaths. No generally satisfactory explanation as to the cause of these adverse reactions has been advanced. Many thousands, perhaps millions, of dogs have been vaccinated with no untoward effect from the vaccine itself, and there is no doubt that vaccination has in many instances been unjustly accused of causing trouble for which it was in no way responsible. Since there is a possibility of a negative phase following vaccination (a period in which an animal might be sensitive to infection preceding the establishment of immunity), it is desirable to confine treated dogs in such a manner as to avoid the possibility of exposure for 2 to 3 weeks.

Much experimental work on rabies has been done in recent years, and laboratory methods for the evaluation of rabies vaccine have been made available. By their use it is now possible to produce more uniformly potent rabies vaccines than were available in the past. On the basis of the recent experimental work, the Bureau of Animal Industry now requires that all rabies vaccines prepared by licensed establishments must pass the standards of a test devised by the National Institute of Health.

Need for Public Interest

Table 1 shows that there were at least 9,412 cases of rabies in domestic animals and man in 1938 and 8,314 in 1939. Since the disease once contracted is fatal, much anxiety is caused to persons exposed to rabid or suspected animals. Local treatment of wounds and the necessity of taking anti-rabies treatment, which is expensive, make the presence of rabies in a community a heavy expense. The number of persons who have to take the anti-rabies treatment in this country runs into the thousands annually. In addition to the public-health aspect of the disease, losses of livestock from rabies run into considerable figures annually. As an example of this, the statement is made in a circular issued by one of the Southern States that in 1936 reports from county agents in 105 counties of the State show that the value of livestock lost from rabies was $65,000 in that State.

It may be noted from Table 1 that rabies does not exist or is of little importance in some States, whereas in many others it is prevalent. In many parts of the country where the disease prevails, misunderstanding concerning its nature and the efforts made to control it has resulted in dissension which has hampered control measures. Probably, however, one of the most important reasons for the prevalence of rabies in many sections is the lack of funds to carry out the control measures properly.

It is time for the public at large to realize that rabies should be brought under control, with the goal of eventual eradication from the country, and to lend whole-hearted support to control efforts in each community. Once the disease has been eradicated from this country, its reappearance could be prevented by a 6-months quarantine of all dogs imported into the United States from countries where rabies is prevalent.

Chapter 2

DISTEMPER OF DOGS

C.D. Stein[1]

[1] *C.D. Stein is Veterinarian, Pathological Division, Bureau of Animal Industry.*

One of the most common and frequently fatal diseases of young dogs, distemper stin causes many deaths every year, though it can now be largely prevented by vaccination.

Canine Distemper is an acute, highly contagious febrile disease caused by a filtrable virus and affecting principally young dogs. The disease is characterized by a catarrhal inflammation of all the mucous membranes of the body, which is frequently accompanied by nervous symptoms and pustular eruptions of the skin. It has its human counterpart in the form of influenza, which, though not identical with distemper, is very similar in many respects.

This insidious disease, which has been referred to by some writers as the "scourge of dogdom," is one of the most common and fatal diseases affecting dogs and has probably been the subject of more discussion and investigation than any other canine malady.

It will be readily appreciated from the foregoing that distemper is a very serious and complicated disease, requiring expert attention; hence, when a dog is suspected of having it, a veterinarian should be consulted immediately. However, persons who have some knowledge of the general characteristics and methods of prevention and control of the disease are in a position to reduce to a minimum the danger that their dogs will acquire it and to safeguard affected dogs, at least to some extent, from its ravages and after effects. The purpose of this discussion is to furnish such information rather than to outline a thorough course of treatment for distemper.

Distemper is known in all countries where there are dogs and occurs in all parts of the United States at all seasons of the year, but it appears to be more prevalent during the winter and the cold damp weather of early spring and late autumn. While young dogs of all breeds are susceptible, it appears to be more common in highly bred animals than in mongrels. Puppies with weak constitutions, and pampered, overfed, under-exercised pet dogs kept in overheated quarters appear to contract the infection more readily and suffer more from the disease than hardy animals properly fed and living in a natural environment.

While distemper is, as stated, primarily a disease of young dogs, affecting principally animals between the ages of 2 months and 1 year, typical cases are occasionally observed in mature dogs. The disease rarely occurs in unweaned pups, since some degree of protection is passed on to a nursing litter through the milk of the bitch.

According to Kirk[2] distemper is most prevalent during the process of dentition, occurring most commonly in puppies 6 weeks to 9 months old, but cases have been observed in pups as young as 10 to 14 days old and in rare instances in very old dogs.

Few species of animals other than dogs are susceptible to the disease. Cats, rabbits, guinea pigs, rats, and human beings are not susceptible. The ferret is extremely susceptible and is used as a laboratory animal by research workers in studying the disease. Reports indicate that distemper may occur in minks, weasels, foxes, wolves, wild dogs, lynxes, and raccoons in captivity.

Devitalising influences which decrease the resistance of puppies, such as rickets, parasitic infestation, insanitary, poorly ventilated kennels, lack of exercise, and an unbalanced diet, are factors predisposing to distemper.

---

[2] KIRK, HAMILTON. CANINE DISTEMPER, ITS COMPLICATIONS, SEQUELE, AND TREATMENT. 226 pp., illus. London. 1922.

Cause and Transmission

The primary causative agent was first demonstrated to be a filtrable virus by Carre[3] in 1905. Laidlaw and Dunkin,[4] during their classical researches on this disease in 1926 to 1928, proved conclusively that the primary causative factor in simple, uncomplicated distemper was a filterable virus. This finding has since been confirmed by a number of investigators in this country.

From a clinical standpoint, however, the disease may be divided into a primary filterable virus stage and a secondary stage complicated by invasion of bacterial organisms. Two distinct factors, therefore, play a part in canine distemper: (1) The specific filtrable virus, which produces the early symptoms, and (2) the bacterial organisms, such as *Alcaligenes bronchisepticus* and others referred to as secondary invaders, which produce serious complicating conditions usually associated with the disease. In this respect, distemper in dogs is analogous to influenza in horses, swine, and human beings, in which a specific virus plays the primary and bacterial organisms a secondary role.

The virus is readily destroyed by heat and by most of the common disinfectants in a few hours, but it resists drying and low temperatures for several days. At temperatures below freezing it can survive for months.

Although it is often impossible to ascertain the source of infection in outbreaks of distemper in individual dogs or kennels, it is known that the infection may spread from affected to susceptible animals either by direct or indirect contact. Where large numbers of dogs are assembled, as in dog pounds, shows, pet shops, or boarding kennels, the infection is apt to exist and be spread to susceptible dogs. According to Laidlaw and Dunkin, distemper is highly infectious in the early stages, even before clinical symptoms are noticeable. They further reported that the virus was uniformly found in the nasal secretion and blood early in the disease but not always late in the attack. There was also evidence that infection might be carried short distances in the air in confined places.

---

3 CARRE. H. SUR LA MALADIE DES JEUNES CHIENS. [Paris] Acad. des Sci. Compt. Rend. 140: 689-690. 1905.

4 LAIDLAW, P.P., and DUNKIN, G.W. A REPORT UPON THE CAUSE AND PREVENTION OF DOG DISTEMPER. Vet. Jour. 84: 600-637. illus. 1928.

Pyle[5] regards droplet infection as the principal factor in natural transmission. In transmission experiments with ferrets he was unable to demonstrate that the infection was air-borne. In further experiments with dogs he obtained evidence to indicate that animals that had recovered from distemper or those immunized with live virus were not virus carriers.

Symptoms and Diagnosis

The period of incubation in distemper (that is, the length of time between exposure to infection and the appearance of the first symptoms), is very variable. Laidlaw and Dunkin reported that under experimental conditions the incubation period tends to be constant at 4 days, with a minimum of 3 days and a maximum of 6. Pyle regards 4 or 5 days as the average period of incubation. Regenos[6] considers the incubation period from natural exposure to range from 4 to 10 days or longer, with an average of about a week. He further reports that the average course of the disease, whether it ends in recovery or death, is 29 days, while seriously complicated cases may run a course of 4 to 12 weeks. Dailey[7], in reporting on observations made on more than 3,600 cases in 1 year, states that in natural exposure the incubation period is about 7 days and that the disease runs a course of about 4 weeks, barring complications.

The symptoms in an established case of distemper depends to a large extent on the form the disease takes and are therefore very variable.

The early symptoms as a rule, are of so mild a nature that they are recognized by careful observers only. These first symptoms may be a rise in the body temperature and watery discharges from the eyes and nose. The appetite may be somewhat impaired, and the general disposition becomes more or less sluggish. In about a week's time the symptoms become well marked, a discharge of mucus and pus from eyes and nose appears, and complications of a more or

---

[5] PYLE, NORMAN J. CANINE DISTEMPER AND ITS BIOLOGICAL THERAPY. Vet. Med. 29: 116-119. 1934.

[6] REGENOS, S.H. CANINE DISTEMPER AND ITS CONTROL. Amer. Vet. Med. Assoc. Jour. 86: 84-95. 1935.

[7] DAILEY, HUGH F. CANINE DISTEMPER. Pa. Univ. School Vet. Med., Vet. Ext. Quart. 29 (29): 1-7. 1929.

less serious nature, such as broncho-pneumonia, hemorrhagic inflammation of the gastrointestinal tract, and disturbances of the brain and spinal cord, frequently set in. During the early stages of the disease, the body temperature may suddenly rise from the normal 101° F. to 103° or 105°. Shivering, dryness of the nostrils and a slight dry cough, increased thirst, a drowsy expression of the eyes, and a desire to sleep may be observed. Later diarrhoea, pneumonia, convulsions, paralysis, or chorea (a nervous disorder) may develop. An inflammation of the membranes of the eyes may sometimes occur, which in turn may permanently damage the eyesight through ulceration or opacity of the cornea. Extreme weakness and a great loss of body weight occur in the advanced stages.

The changes in the body tissues resulting from canine distemper, like the clinical symptoms, are variable. In acute uncomplicated cases, enlargement of the spleen and abdominal lymph glands and the presence of a few scattered pin-point hemorrhages may constitute the only lesions, or tissue alterations. Subacute and chronic cases usually cause marked alterations in the respiratory and gastrointestinal tracts due to bacterial infection with secondary invaders. Hemorrhagic areas, congestion, edema (watery swelling), or pneumonia may be observed in the lungs, whereas a catarrhal or hemorrhagic enteritis, or intestinal inflammation, and exudates in the abdominal cavity may also be found.

On account of its obscure nature and great similarity to other catarrhal affections of bacterial origin, the diagnosis of distemper is sometimes difficult, especially in the early stages. In young dogs with a history of exposure to the disease, however, an elevation of body temperature, together with shivering, sneezing, partial loss of appetite, a slight eye and nasal discharge, sluggishness, and diarrhoea, is very suggestive of distemper.

Treatment and Prevention

Good nursing and proper care are important in promoting the recovery of sick dogs. Like similar febrile diseases due to filtrable viruses, distemper runs a definite course regardless of any medicinal treatment that may be administered. Therefore, nostrums advanced as so-called quick cures for distemper have no value.

The treatment of distemper is largely concerned with alleviating the symptoms and is usually attended with considerable difficulty.

No drug or combination of drugs is known at this time that has a specific action in this disease. Homologous anti-canine-distemper serum, a biological product prepared from the blood of immune dogs that have been hyper immunized against the disease, is of value in lessening the severity of an attack if administered subcutaneously or intravenously (under the skin or into the veins) during the early stages of the disease. Dogs affected with distemper should be provided with clean, warm, dry, well-ventilated quarters and should be given only small quantities of such easily digested, nourishing foods as milk, raw eggs, raw beef, and beef broth. Affected animals should be kept quiet and can be kept clean by daily grooming with brush and comb. The eyes and nose should be kept free from accumulated discharges. The eyes may be bathed with a weak boric acid solution to allay irritation, and petrolatum may be applied to the edges of the nostrils to prevent cracking and irritation of the skin. Under no circumstances should an affected animal be permitted to get wet or chilled, nor should drugs be administered unless prescribed by a veterinarian. When the animal begins to show signs of improvement it must not be given an undue quantity of food at one meal, since overeating may cause a relapse or even death. The convalescing dog should be allowed to exercise only very moderately.

Diseases of the nervous system frequently occur during or after an attack of distemper. Chorea, a disease characterized by a persistent twitching of certain muscles or groups of muscles, is one of the most common of these affections. No specific treatment can be recommended to cure chorea. There is a tendency for the twitching to become progressively worse and terminate in paralysis of one or more groups of muscles. A nutritious diet of fresh meat, milk, and eggs, regular evacuation of the bowels and bladder, and clean, warm, dry, and comfortable surroundings free from annoyance may assist in the recovery of mild cases. The treatment of the after effects of distemper, like that of the disease itself, should be under the supervision of a qualified veterinarian.

Much progress has been made in recent years in immunization against canine distemper, but in spite of the great advances made in the control of the disease, it still takes a heavy annual death toll among unvaccinated dogs and causes considerable financial losses to owners and breeders.

There are two recognized standard methods of distemper prophylaxis, or prevention: (1) The vaccine-virus, or Laidlaw-Dunkin method, which consists in the administration of vaccine followed by living virus and (2) the serum-virus method, which consists in the administration of anti-canine-distemper serum and living virus. The different methods of vaccination now in use in this country are all modifications of one or the other of these basic forms of immunization. The Department of Agriculture has conducted no tests to determine the relative merits of the different methods of immunization, but reports from the field indicate that, when properly applied, any one is an effective means of controlling the disease.

It is generally believed that puppies should not be immunized against distemper until they are at least 3 months old. Some investigators who have done considerable research on this problem are of the opinion that when puppies under 4 to 6 months of age are vaccinated, complete immunity is not produced. When danger of infection is imminent, however, puppies 6 to 8 weeks old may be protected by the administration of vaccine or anti-canine-distemper serum and revaccinated at 4 to 6 months of age by one of the standard methods of immunization, which should include the administration of living virus. The dog to be vaccinated should be free from parasites and rickets and in a state of general good health.

The vaccination of dogs against distemper should be undertaken only by a qualified veterinarian, as proper immunization involves not only an understanding of the principles of immunity but the consideration of a number of other factors.

In the control of distemper it is important that affected animals be promptly isolated, as close contact between infected and susceptible dogs during an outbreak results in a rapid passage of the disease to the latter.

Inasmuch as distemper is caused by a specific contagion that is known to remain alive and active outside the animal body, it is essential that after an outbreak the premises be thoroughly disinfected before susceptible animals are brought in. For this purpose, a 5-percent solution of phenol, a 2-percent formaldehyde solution, a 2-percent lye solution, or a 3-percent compound solution of cresol, U.S.P. may be used.

To eradicate completely the contagion of distemper from the premises, it is essential that all objects that have come in contact with affected dogs, as well as the quarters occupied by them, be thoroughly cleaned and disinfected. All litter or old bedding should be burned. The infective agent is destroyed in a short time when exposed to direct sunlight. It would be advisable to allow several weeks to elapse even after a thorough cleansing and disinfection of the premises before bringing in a new puppy, unless the puppy has previously been immunized against distemper.

Chapter 3

FELINE ENTERITIS

C.D. Stein [1]

[1] *C. D. Stein is Veterinarian, Pathological Division, Bureau of Animal Industry.*

In its disastrous effects on young animals and its high mortality rate, feline enteritis is the counterpart of distemper of dogs. Here is a description of the disease and an account of such control measures as are available.

Feline Enteritis is an acute, specific, infectious, highly contagious disease of cats, usually young cats, commonly known as infectious gastroenteritis and feline distemper.[2] It is also referred to as croupous enteritis, epizootic enteritis, malignant panleucopenia, infectious feline agranulocytosis, and feline typhus. The disease, which is world-wide in distribution, occurs in all parts of the United States in cats of all breeds and at all seasons, but it appears to be most prevalent during the cold damp weather of early spring and late autumn. It is considered to be the most serious disease

[2] The term, "feline distemper" is also used to designate a mild infectious disease of young cats, characterized by catarrhal inflammation of the mucous membranes, known as feline influenza. Kirk (*5*)[3] and Salsbery (*10*) consider feline distemper to be an entirely distinct disease. Hindle and Findlay (*4*), on the other hand, describe an infectious disease of cats due to a filtrable virus with symptoms similar to feline infectious enteritis as feline distemper.

[3] Italic numbers in parentheses refer to Literature Cited.

encountered in cats and takes its greatest death toll among kittens and young cats. It often occurs as an epizootic (corresponding to an epidemic among human beings) affecting and rapidly decimating the entire young cat population in certain districts. The occurrence of the disease has recently been reported by Torres (*11*) in wild as well as domestic cats in Brazil.

Feline enteritis is characterized principally by its sudden onset, highly contagious nature, rapid and violent course, profound alterations in the blood, and frequent fatal termination, and by its predilection for young cats. Although the symptoms are variable, those most characteristic are high fever, loss of appetite, enteritis (acute inflammation of the intestinal tract), a marked decrease of white blood cells, rapid loss of flesh, great depression, diarrhoea, vomiting, and sometimes a discharge from the eyes and nose. Affected cats manifest extreme soreness of the abdomen and may assume a peculiar characteristic position, lying flat on the abdomen with head lowered, forelegs spread laterally, and hind legs stretched out. Roughening of the coat, complete loss of appetite, sudden elevation of temperature, and depression are usually the first symptoms observed. These may be followed by severe diarrhoea, the stool sometimes being streaked with blood, vomiting, extreme weakness, marked emaciation, complete exhaustion, and death.

The incubation period, that is, the time between exposure to the infection and the appearance of the first symptoms, is 5 to 6 days under experimental conditions and 6 to 8 days or longer in natural infection. The course of the disease is usually very rapid, affected animals sometimes dying in 24 to 48 hours, and in especially acute cases, particularly in kittens, it is often so rapid that death may occur before any well-marked symptoms develop. Cases of this type, particularly when several cats in the same neighbourhood are similarly affected, are frequently mistaken by the owners for poisoning. The mortality is high, often exceeding 80 percent.

As a rule definite lesions, or tissue alterations, mainly in the intestinal tract, are observed on post mortem examination, though in some cases such lesions may be slight or lacking. Inflammation of the small and large intestines is usually present, varying in intensity from simple congestion to a well-marked hemorrhagic enteritis involving all or a portion of the intestinal tract. The mesenteric lymph glands (in the intestinal region) may be congested and show an infiltration of blood due to hemorrhages. Moderate congestion of the liver, spleen, and kidneys may also be observed in some cases.

Devitalizing influences that decrease the resistance of kittens, such as rickets, parasitic infestation (particularly hookworms), insanitary, poorly ventilated quarters, and under-nourishment, are predisposing factors to feline infectious enteritis.

The causative agent is a filtrable virus. Verge and Cristoforoni (*13*) in 1928 were the first to establish this fact, and others have confirmed the finding.[4]

A highly infectious and acute disease of young cats, due to a filtrable virus, characterized by marked changes in the blood, with clinical symptoms of enteritis, and considered to be identical with feline enteritis, has been described under different names by various investigators,[5] all of whom have pointed out that in addition to enteritis, leucopenia (a decrease in the white blood cells) is a more or less constant finding of considerable diagnostic importance in this disease.

As already noted, the disease frequently occurs as an epizootic and is so highly contagious that it spreads rapidly when once established. Natural infection may occur by direct contact of healthy with diseased cats or by exposure to contaminated quarters, bedding, utensils, or other articles that have been in contact with infected cats. Macchiavello and Bezerra Coutinho (*9*) were the first workers to present evidence that fleas may harbour the virus, and recently Torres (*11*) reported evidence definitely indicating that fleas may play an important role in the spread of the disease.

According to Leasure, Lienhardt, and Taberner (*8*), who made an extensive study of this disease, the virus is found in the urine, feces, and blood and remains alive for a considerable length of time. They reported that virus kept under refrigeration at 42° F. and also

---

[4] Hindle and Findley (*4*) in 1932, Urban (*12*) in 1933, Leasure, Lienhardt, and Taberner (*8*) in 1934, and Salsbery (*10*) in 1938.

[5] By Macchiavello and Bezerra Countinho (*9*) as infectious adenomyeloenterosis; by Lawrence and Syverton (*6*) as spontaneous agranulocytosis; by Lawrence, Syverton, Shaw, and Smith (*7*) as infectious agranulocytosis; by Hammon and Enders (*2, 3*) as malignant panleucopenia; and by Torres (*11*) as feline gastroenteritis.

virus kept at room temperature (50° to 85° F.) remained virulent for 91 days.

The successful immunization of cats against this disease under experimental conditions, either by the use of tissue vaccine treated with formalin (formalized) prepared from the organs of infected cats or by the simultaneous injection of feline infectious enteritis virus and homologous hyperimmune antiserum (prepared with material from cats), has been reported.[6] As a result of studies on immunization against malignant panleucopenia (now considered identical with feline infectious enteritis), Enders and Hammon (*1*) reported evidence to indicate that resistance to the disease in susceptible cats can be induced by the injection of formalized suspensions of organs from infected cats. They also reported that the serum of cats that have recovered from the infection, as well as that of animals immunized against the disease, will protect susceptible cats for a limited time against subsequent exposure. Biological products (vaccines, antisera, and bacterins) are commercially available for use in the treatment and prevention of the disease. While the Department of Agriculture has carried on no experiments to determine the relative merits of these products, reports from the practicing veterinarians indicate that these biologics may have some value if properly applied.

From the field of small-animal practice it has been reported that:

(1) Improvement is often noted in sick cats following the administration of repeated large doses of homologous feline enteritis serum and that the administration of such serum is the best prophylactic (preventive) measure for healthy cats during an epidemic of the disease.

(2) If treatment with serum is commenced in the early stages of the disease before the temperature begins to drop, a large percentage of cases can be saved. For best results, treatment with a combination of homologous feline enteritis antiserum injected into the abdominal cavity and mixed antibacterial feline serum injected under the skin is recommended.

(3) Complete protection of young kittens against the disease during hospital exposure can be assured by prophylactic

[6] By Urbain (*12*), Leasnre, Lienhardt, and Taberner (*8*), and Salsbery (*10*).

doses of 2 to 3 cubic centimetres of serum obtained from immune adult cats that have been exposed to the disease.

No specific medicinal treatment is known for this disease. Affected cats should be isolated and placed in warm, dry quarters. If animals show an inclination to take nourishment, a diet of broth, milk, and raw eggs should be supplied. The administration of biologics and drugs for the treatment and relief of affected cats should be undertaken only by a qualified veterinarian.

In controlling outbreaks of the disease, immediate isolation of sick animals from healthy ones and a prompt and thorough cleaning and disinfection of premises are of first importance. To prevent new cats brought into the house from acquiring infectious enteritis after an outbreak, it is necessary to eradicate the infection from the premises. To accomplish this, it is essential that all objects that have come in contact with diseased cats, as well as the quarters occupied by them, be thoroughly cleaned and disinfected. All litter and bedding should be burned. A period of at least 2 to 3 months should elapse before restocking with healthy cats.

Since it has been definitely shown that fleas may transmit the disease from infected to susceptible cats, necessary steps should also be taken to eliminate flea infestation, both in the house and on cats.

Literature Cited

(1) ENDERS, JOHN F., and HAMMON, WILLIAM D. (1940). ACTIVE AND PASSIVE IMMUNIZATION AGAINST THE VIRUS OF MALIGNANT PANLEUCOPENIA OF CATS. Soc. Expt. Biol. and Med. Proc. 43: 194-200.

(2) HAMMON, WILLIAM D., and ENDERS, JOHN F. (1939). A VIRUS DISEASE OF CATS, PRINCIPALLY CHARACTERIZED BY ALEUCOCYTOSIS, ENTERIC LESIONS AND THE PRESENCE OF INTRANUCLEAR INCLUSION BODIES. Jour. Expt. Med. 69: 327-352, illus.

(3) ______and ENDERS, JOHN F. (1939). FURTHER STUDIES ON THE BLOOD AND THE HEMATOPOIETIC TISSUES IN MALIGNANT PANLEUCOPENIA OF CATS. Jour. Expt. Med. 70: 557-564, illus.

(4) HINDLE, E., and FINDLAY, G.M. (1932). STUDIES ON FELINE DISTEMPER. Jour. Compar. Path. and Ther. 45: 11-26.

(5) KIRK, HAMILTON (1933). FELINE DISTEMPER VERSUS SPECIFIC FELINE INFECTIOUS ENTERITIS. Vet. Rec. 45: [147]-149.

(6) LAWRENCE, JOHN S., and SYVERTON, JEROME T. (1938). SPONTANEOUS AGRANULOCYTOSIS IN THE CAT. Soc. Expt. Biol. and Med. Proc. 38: 914-918, illus.

(7) _____SYVERTON, JEROME T., SHAW, JOHN S., and SMITH, FRANK P. (1940). INFECTIOUS FELINE AGRANULOCYTOSIS. Amer. Jour. Path. 16: 333-354, illus.

(8) LEASURE, E.E., LIENHARDT, H.F., and TABERNER, F.R. (1934). FELINE INFECTIOUS ENTERITIS. North Amer. Vet. 15 (7): 30-44, illus.

(9) MACCHIAVELLO, ATILIO, and COUTINHO, ALUZIO BEZERRA (1940). EPIZOOTIAS FELINAS DO NORDESTE DO BBASIL ADENO-MYELOENTEROSE ESPECIPIA POR VIRUS FILTRAVEL. [FELINE DISEASES IN THE NORTH-EAST OF BRAZIL]. Brazil Med. 54: [113]-118.

(10) SALSBERY, C.E. (1939). INFECTIOUS GASTROENTERITIS OF CATS. Amer. Vet. Med. Assoc. Jour. 95: 195-200.

(11) TORRES, SYLVIO (1941). INFECTIOUS FELINE GASTROENTERITIS IN WILD CATS. North Amer. Vet. 22: 297-299.

(12) URBAIN, ACH (1933). CONTRIBUTION A L'ETUDE DE LA GASTRO-ENTERITE INFECTIEUSE DES CHATS. Ann de l'Inst. Pasteur 51: 202-214.

(18) VERGE, J., and CRISTOFORONI, N. (1928). LA GASTRO-ENTERITE INFECTIEUSE DES CHATS: EST-ELLE DUE A UN VIRUS FILTRABLE? Soc. de Biol. [Paris] Compt. Rend. 99: 312-314.

Chapter 4

MISCELLANEOUS DISEASES OF DOGS AND CATS

C.D. Stein [1]

[1] *C.D. Stein is Veterinarian, Pathological Division, Bureau of Animal Industry.*

Condensed facts and suggestions concerning a host of conditions about which the pet owner should have some knowledge.

Keeping pet animals well depends largely on giving them intelligent care. Hence proper and regular feeding, sufficient and regular exercise, hygienic surroundings, warm, dry, well-ventilated sleeping quarters, provision for regular evacuation of the bowels and bladder, freedom from parasitic infestation, and regular and proper grooming are extremely important. Observance of these recognized commonsense methods of management, together with an elementary knowledge of the causes and characteristics of the common ailments, will materially assist pet owners in maintaining their animals in good condition and safeguarding them against many of the common maladies.

The home treatment of ailments of pet animals with so-called "sure-cure" remedies is frequently dangerous, since many diseases are of a serious nature and require expert attention. It is therefore suggested that, when possible, treatment should be under the supervision of a veterinarian specializing in diseases of small pet animals.

Abnormal Growths

Abnormal growths in dogs and cats may be due to the formation of abscesses, cysts, or tumors, to the enlargement of superficial glands, or to hernias.

An abscess is an enlargement due to an accumulation of pus enclosed in a capsule and may occur on any part of the body. It frequently follows injuries such as scratches, bites, and puncture wounds which permit pus-producing micoorganisms to enter the tissues.

Pain in the area of the abscess, caused by pressure on the tissues, and a rise in body temperature may occur. Treatment consists in the use of hot applications to bring the abscess to a head, an incision with a sterile knife at the lowest point for drainage, and the application of mild antiseptics.

A cyst is a fluctuating tumorlike enlargement due to the accumulation and distention of tissue cavities with a fluid or semifluid substance.

There are a number of different types of cysts, but the most common in the dog and cat is the blood cyst of the ear (haematoma), which follows an injury. Cysts of other types may occur in the skin on different parts of the body, on the eyelids, in the ovaries, and in the uterus. Since surgical interference is indicated in most types of cysts, the diagnosis and treatment of this condition should be left to a veterinarian.

Tumors are enlargements due to tissue growth of a morbid nature. They may appear in any part of the body and occur for the most part in aged animals–for example, tumors of the mammary gland in old female dogs and skin tumors in old cats. Tumors are of two types–malignant tumors, which develop rapidly and may spread progressively to other tissues in the body and destroy them; and non-malignant tumors, which grow slowly and are usually well encapsulated, or enclosed in a surrounding membrane. Non-malignant tumors occasionally become malignant, but as a rule they remain localized, though they may grow to a large size and interfere with the functions of the parts affected. Early diagnosis and surgical removal of tumors are important, and for this reason a veterinarian should be consulted immediately if their presence is suspected.

Mumps (parotitis) is an enlargement and inflammation of the salivary glands due to injury or infection. The affection manifests itself by a rapidly developing swelling of the glands and surrounding tissues of the ear. The head and neck may become enlarged, swallowing may be difficult, fever develops, and abscesses may form in the affected glands. Affected dogs should be isolated, and treatment should be under the supervision of a veterinarian.

Goiter is an enlargement of the thyroid gland and appears as a swelling on both sides of the trachea (windpipe) in the lower part of the neck. In some cases the glands become greatly enlarged, making breathing difficult. Daily applications of tincture of iodine externally for 4 or 5 days are sometimes beneficial. Good results have also been reported from administering thyroid extract.

Hodgkins disease (lymphadenoma) is marked by enlargement of the lymphatic glands in various parts of the body. The cause of the disease is not definitely known, and no satisfactory treatment has been discovered.

Rupture (hernia) may be described as a saclike enlargement in the abdominal wall produced by the protrusion of abdominal organs (principally the intestines) through a small opening in the wall into the surrounding tissues. There are several different types of rupture that take their name from the structures affected. Umbilical, abdominal, scrotal, and inguinal (groin) ruptures are the most common in the cat and dog. Hereditary or acquired defects in the abdominal wall and increased abdominal pressure are the direct causes of rupture. Enlargements in the region of the abdomen caused by abscesses and tumors may be mistaken for rupture. Diagnosis and treatment should be left to a veterinarian.

Anal Gland Infection

The anal glands in the dog, located in each side of the rectum near its terminal point, normally secrete a grayish-brown substance with a fetid odour. The opening in the glands sometimes becomes clogged, especially in old dogs, resulting in sensitive swellings on both sides of the rectum at the margin of the anus. Affected animals show evidences of pain on defecation, drag themselves on the floor, and lick and bite at the rectum. In mild cases the condition can be relieved by squeezing out the glands by pressing them between the thumb and forefinger. In cases of long standing, the formation of pus, accompanied by an abscess, often occurs, requiring surgical treatment.

Ascites (Dropsy)

Ascites is characterized by the collection of fluid in the abdominal cavity, which causes it to become enlarged and pendulous. It is usually the result of disease conditions affecting the heart, liver, or kidneys, and is most often seen in old dogs. Treatment is not very satisfactory. The condition can be relieved by puncturing and draining off fluid, but the trouble tends to recur. Treatment should be under the supervision of a veterinarian.

Ailments of Aged Dogs

Instances are on record which show that in exceptional cases, dogs may live 20 years or longer. The average life of dogs, however, is generally considered to be from 10 to 12 years. Old or aging dogs are subject to a number of afflictions, such as asthma, ascites, diseases of the heart, liver, and kidneys, cataracts, deafness, arthritis, and toxemia, or general poisoning of the system.

In the aged dog, little can be done to cure these conditions, but good care, comfortable quarters, a pleasant environment, and nourishing, easily digested food, together with persistent treatment for the relief of chronic ailments, will materially assist in prolonging the life of the animal.

Blacktongue

Blacktongue is sometimes mistaken for or referred to as canine typhus, Stuttgart disease, or hemorrhagic gastroenteritis (inflammation of the stomach and intestines). It is an acute, often fatal disease characterized by a severe stomatitis, or inflammation of the mouth, and gastroenteritis.

The disease may affect young dogs but is most common in middle age or old age. It is considered to be a nutritional disease. Experimental evidence indicates that a diet deficient in nicotinic acid and perhaps other B vitamins is probably the cause.

The first symptom usually observed in affected animals is inflammation of the membranes of the mouth, accompanied by drooling. In a short time the inflamed areas on the lips, gums, and tongue ulcerate and slough away, and the tongue may assume a bluish-black colour, which gives the disease its name. The mouth has a characteristic putrid odour. Loss of appetite, frequent vomiting, a bloody, fetid diarrhoea, a rapid loss of weight due to loss of water from the tissues (dehydration), and great weakness are manifested during the rapid course of the disease.

Dietary treatment is of first importance in its prevention and cure. If it has not progressed too far, the disease will usually respond to treatment with pure dried yeast, ½ to 1 ounce, depending on the size of the dog, given two or three times daily, plus well-balanced rations. In addition to dried yeast, fresh meat, fresh milk, canned salmon, and liver are highly effective in the prevention and treatment of blacktongue, while fresh eggs, tomato juice, and whole-wheat products furnish protection to a somewhat less extent.

Digestive Disorders

Diseases of the digestive tract, usually due to improper feeding, are among the most common ailments of dogs and cats.

Vomiting, diarrhoea, and constipation are the common symptoms in ordinary digestive disorders, but they may also occur in a number of specific diseases. Mild attacks of vomiting and diarrhoea, and constipation when it has not lasted too long, may frequently be cleared up by the removal from the digestive tract of irritant substances, or hardened fecal matter in the case of constipation, through the administration of suitable purgatives such as mineral oil, milk of magnesia, or castor oil, or the use of enemas. Affected animals should be placed on a diet of nourishing, easily digested foods, such as boiled skimmed milk, egg yolks, gruels, meat broth free from excessive fat, ground fresh lean beef, and small amounts of gelatin. The addition of small amounts of limewater, boiled rice, or barley and cheese to the diet may help to check mild cases of diarrhoea, and the administration of bismuth subnitrate is also of value.

Perverted appetite in pet animals, that is, the eating of dirt, fecal matter, and other indigestible materials, may be due to a deficiency of certain minerals in the diet or to a deficiency of vitamins, to parasitic infestation, or to habit. Grass eating is also a habit acquired by some dogs and is observed when there are digestive disorders or thirst, and in sultry weather. Animals showing signs of a depraved appetite should be kept in clean quarters, fed a balanced ration containing meat and milk, and given plenty of exercise. Small amounts of limewater, calcium lactate, cod-liver oil, and yeast in the diet are also of value.

Pet animals, especially dogs, are apt to swallow sharp objects such as pins, needles, tacks, fishhooks, and other things which may lodge in the tongue, esophagus, stomach, or intestines. Bones from chicken, fish, chops, or steaks may also become lodged in the throat and choke the animal. A foreign body produces irritation and inflammation at the point of lodgment; its exact location should be determined, and it should be removed by a veterinarian.

Concretions of hair, known as hair balls, sometimes form in the intestines of cats owing to continual swallowing of hair. Hair balls sometimes become quite large, producing digestive disturbances and at times fecal impaction. Daily grooming of long-haired cats and of short-haired ones during shedding will help to prevent this trouble.

A common trouble of both dogs and cats is due directly to the consumption of indigestible material which obstructs the intestine. The symptoms include loss of appetite, vomiting, distention and rigidity of the abdomen, and constipation. Intestinal irrigation and the administration of mineral oil for removal of the foreign material, followed by a liquid diet, is the usual treatment.

Gastroenteritis, an inflammation of the mucous membrane (lining) of the stomach and intestines, is a common malady in pet animals, especially dogs.

There are two types, a catarrhal and a hemorrhagic form.

The catarrhal form may run an acute or chronic course and is due principally to improper feeding. Other causative factors are swallowing decomposed food, indigestible material, and chemical poisons, as well as parasitic infestation and bacterial infection. Affected animals may show a decrease in appetite, increased thirst, tenderness and pain in the region of the stomach, general uneasiness, and some stiffness in moving about and may vomit frequently. In severe cases, diarrhoea may develop. If not corrected, repeated attacks of acute catarrhal gastritis may develop into the chronic form.

Since faulty feeding is usually the cause of this condition, the treatment is principally dietetic. In mild cases, food should be withheld for a day or two, and purgatives such as milk of magnesia or castor oil should be administered to eliminate irritants from the digestive tract. The diet should consist of small quantities of easily digested foods such as milk, eggs, beef extract, gelatin, and later ground fresh lean beef. Chronic cases in which there is frequent vomiting may require irrigation of the stomach with a weak solution of sodium bicarbonate, together with other special treatment by a veterinarian.

Hemorrhagic gastroenteritis is an acute inflammation of the lining of the stomach and intestines with a discharge of blood (hemorrhage) into the intestinal tract. The causes are the same as those given for the catarrhal form. Hemorrhagic gastroenteritis may also occur as one of the principal symptoms in different types of poisoning and in a number of specific diseases of the dog such as blacktongue, distemper, and infectious leptospirosis, as well as in infectious feline enteritis of cats.

The symptoms observed in affected animals are loss of appetite, vomiting, increased thirst, foul breath, abdominal pain, bloody diarrhoea, rapid loss of flesh, dehydration, and extreme weakness.

Since this is a serious disease that usually runs a rapid course, the diagnosis and treatment should be left to a veterinarian.

Ear Diseases

The two most common ear affections in the dog and cat are otorrhea (canker) and haematoma.

The two types of ear canker are: (1) External canker, characterized by ulceration of the concha (lobe) and edges of the external ear, and (2) internal canker, which may be of parasitic or non-parasitic origin, characterized by inflammation and infection of the ear canal. Frequent shaking of the head and scratching the ear with the paws are indicative of ear affections.

Dogs with long ears, such as hounds and setters, are most frequently affected with external canker, which is caused by injuries to the ear such as cuts, scratches, and bites, which later become infected. The constant shaking of the head and scratching of the ear, together with fly bites, increase the irritation and tend to prevent healing. When of long standing, the condition is often resistant to treatment. Cleaning the affected part with soap and water to remove dried crusts, daily application of an antiseptic dusting powder, and protection of the ears against further injury or irritation from fly bites will assist in clearing up mild cases.

In internal canker the ear canal shows inflammation and the formation of pus and produces a profuse brownish-coloured putrid discharge. The condition may be caused by the irritation produced by mange mites or by the accumulation of ear secretions, dirt, and hair, or it may occur as a complication in eczema, distemper, and other diseases.

Daily cleansing of the ear canal with sterile cotton swabs dipped in ether or alcohol, followed by the application of a few drops of 2-percent carbolic acid in sweet oil or glycerin will help to clear up mild cases if treatment is commenced during the early inflammatory stages of the disease before pus has begun to form. Cases of long standing, however, are usually difficult to cure, requiring persistent and painstaking attention over a long period of time; and even then the results are sometimes unsatisfactory. Treatment of these cases should be under the supervision of a veterinarian.

Haematoma of the ear is common in dogs, especially those with long, floppy ears, but occurs less frequently in cats. It appears as a sensitive swelling between the skin and the cartilage of the ear. Haematoma usually develops suddenly and is the result of injuries which rupture small blood vessels, permitting the escape of blood and serum into the tissue spaces between the skin and the cartilage. Treatment is surgical and consists in drawing off the excess fluid, followed by suturing (stitching) and the application of antiseptics.

Eclampsia

Eclampsia is a nervous affection occurring in the nursing bitch and characterized by convulsions. The cause is not definitely known, but the condition is believed by some observers to be associated with a calcium deficiency.[2] It is occasionally observed in pregnant bitches just prior to whelping but most often occurs a few days to several weeks after parturition.

---

[2] For a brief discussion of eclampsia as a nutritional disease.

The attacks appear suddenly. The symptoms are first panting, excitement, and restlessness, soon followed by convulsive spasms; the animal falls on its side and may kick violently. The muscles become tense, breathing is rapid, the pulse is accelerated, mucous membranes are congested, and there is an increased flow of saliva. The animal remains conscious during an attack. The duration and severity of an attack vary, but affected animals should receive immediate treatment.

Intravenous injection of calcium gluconate is the most satisfactory treatment and should be administered by a veterinarian. Administration of sedatives, such as morphine and nembutal, is of value in controlling an acute attack. The affected bitch should be placed in warm, quiet quarters and not allowed to nurse her puppies during the attack or for some time after recovery.

Eye Diseases

The eyes of pet animals, like those of human beings, are subject to many diseases; only the most common ailments will be dealt with in this discussion.

Conjunctivitis, an inflammation of the membranes lining the eyelids, may be caused by irritants, injuries, and infections, or it may be a symptom of certain febrile diseases such as distemper. It manifests itself first by congestion of the membrane and watering of the eyes (lachrymation), followed by formation and discharge of mucus and finally of pus. Frequent washing of the eyes with warm boric acid solution, the application of cold compresses two or three times a day, and placing a drop or two of freshly prepared argyrol (5- to 10-percent solution) or zinc sulfate (1-percent solution) in the eyes will usually clear up this trouble. The application of borated petrolatum to the edges of the eyelids will prevent their being stuck together by the accumulated discharge.

Keratitis is an inflammation of the cornea–the normally transparent covering of the front of the eyeball--due to wounds, the presence of foreign bodies or irritants, or the spread of inflammation from other structures of the eye. It may be mild or serious. The symptoms are lachrymation, photophobia (extreme sensitiveness to light), and clouding of the cornea, indicated by the appearance of a bluish-white film.

The treatment for mild cases is the same as that suggested for conjunctivitis, that is, washing the eyes four or five times daily with warm mild antiseptics, such as boric acid. Severe cases require professional attention.

Suppurative keratitis (ulceration of the cornea) is more or less common in dogs, the ulcers varying in size from pin-point depressions to large, deep, circular or irregular areas. The ulceration may be caused by infection entering through slight wounds, scratches, bites, or other injuries, or it may occur in purulent conjunctivitis and in such infectious diseases as distemper. Inflammation, lachrymation, photophobia, and pus formation are more or less constant symptoms. The healed ulcers frequently leave scars, and this occasionally leads to perforation of the cornea and a permanent opacity. Successful treatment requires professional attention. Flushing out the eye with mild antiseptics, such as 2-percent boric acid, is beneficial and tends to prevent further spread of the ulcer.

Cataract is a disease in which opacity occurs in the lens of the eye and its capsule. Senile cataract is common in aged dogs and cats, but cataract also results from injury and sometimes develops from an attack of distemper. It runs a chronic course, usually ending in loss of vision. Treatment is surgical, but it is frequently unsuccessful and is therefore seldom carried out.

Glaucoma is a disease characterized by marked hardness of the eyeball due to increased tension within the eye. It usually develops slowly, without evidence of inflammation, and causes gradual loss of vision. Treatment is surgical to relieve intraocular pressure but is usually unsatisfactory.

Entropion, an inversion, or turning in, of the eyelids against the cornea, producing inflammation and sometimes ulceration, is common in certain breeds of dogs such as Chows, Spaniels, and Bull Dogs. Ectropion, a turning out of the eyelids, exposing the membranes of the lower lids particularly and causing them to become congested and inflamed with a copious flow of tears, occurs mostly in Setters, Blood-hounds, and Saint Bernards. Application of mild antiseptics will assist in relieving the inflammation of the lids in both these conditions, but surgical procedure is usually necessary to correct the trouble.

Fits (Convulsions or Nervous Spasms)

Common fits, or convulsions, may occur in cats and dogs of all ages but are more common in dogs, especially puppies during teething. A fit is not a disease in itself but merely a symptom of some other disorder, usually of an irritating nature. Violence exercise, nervous excitement, teething in young puppies, indigestion, foreign bodies in the stomach or intestines, parasitic infestation (worms in the intestines or mange mites in the ears) are some of the common causes of fits. They may also occur during the onset of distemper and sometimes appear to be of a hereditary nature (epileptic fits).

Attacks usually occur suddenly; muscular movements become uncontrollable and there is a rigidity affecting all the muscles and champing of the jaws, with the appearance of frothy saliva about the mouth. The animal may finally fall on its side, kick violently, and lose consciousness. After a few minutes, it rises to its feet with a staggering gait and appears to be in a state of bewilderment. When symptoms of a coming seizure are noticed, or during convulsions, the animal should be moved to a quiet, dark room and left alone until it recovers. As a protection against bites and scratches during an attack, a cat or dog should be handled only with heavy gloves or wrapped in a blanket.

After recovery, food should be withheld for a day, and a mild laxative should be given to clear out intestinal-irritants. To prevent further attacks, attempts should be made to determine the source of the trouble.

Icterus (Jaundice or Yellows)

Icterus is a condition characterized by a yellowish discolouration of the skin and the visible mucous membranes, indicative of diseases of the liver interfering with the normal flow of bile.

The two principal types of icterus in the dog are:

(1) A simple or catarrhal form due to obstruction of the bile ducts and occurring in diseases of the liver and in gastric disorders; and

(2) An infectious hemolytic form, known as infectious canine leptospirosis, or sometimes as canine typhus, which is considered to be identical with Weil's disease (infectious jaundice) of human beings.

Infectious canine leptospirosis, while not very prevalent in the United States, has been reported from a number of different localities. The disease occurs in all breeds of dogs but rarely in animals under 8 or 9 months of age. It spreads rapidly and is often fatal. The causative factor is either of two spirochaetes, *Leptospira canicola* or *L. icterohemorrhagiae*, both of which are believed to be carried by rats. There is some evidence that the disease may be transmitted from dogs to man.

Symptoms in affected animals are a high temperature, vomiting, bleeding of the gums, loss of appetite, gastroenteritis, bloody diarrhoea, and frequently jaundice and great depression.

Treatment of this disease is not very satisfactory. Recently, however, antileptospiral serum and vaccine have been used experimentally with very good results. As control measures, steps should be taken to exterminate rats in areas where the disease is known to exist, and the premises where infected dogs have been kept should be cleaned and disinfected.

Metritis

Metritis is an acute or chronic inflammation of the uterus (womb) in the bitch and the female cat, caused by retention of the fatal membranes, infection introduced at the time of parturition, wounds of the mucous membranes of the vagina and uterus, or injuries. Cold, damp kennels are also conducive to the disease. In animals affected with acute metritis there are swelling and congestion of the vulva and vagina with a brownish or blood-stained fetid discharge from the vagina. Other symptoms are fever, loss of appetite, vomiting, and tenderness in the region of the uterus.

Treatment in mild cases consists in irrigation of the uterus with mild antiseptics. In severe cases, surgical treatment is often necessary to effect a cure.

Chronic metritis (pyometra), characterized by the collection of pus in the uterus, occurs more frequently in dogs than in cats and, like the acute form, appears after parturition. It is due to the same causes as the acute form. The principal symptom is the continuous discharge of grayish-red fetid pus from the vulva. Other symptoms are enlargement of the abdomen, emaciation, weakness, and a rough coat.

Treatment is surgical and consists in the removal of the uterus and ovaries.

Posterior Paralysis

Although paralysis of the jaw, forelegs, and groups of muscles in other parts of the body occasionally occurs in the dog, the most common form of paralysis is that of the hind limbs. It may be caused by infectious diseases such as distemper, obscure nervous diseases, injuries to the back, abnormal growths that cause pressure on the spine, intestinal obstructions resulting in autointoxication, heavy infestation by certain types of ticks (tick paralysis), and senility. Weakness or lameness, particularly in puppies, is sometimes mistaken for paralysis.

When paralysis is caused by a toxic infection resulting from obstinate constipation, the condition can frequently be corrected by the use of enemas to clean out the intestinal tract, together with other treatment prescribed by a veterinarian.

A nutritious diet, regular evacuation of the bowels and bladder, and clean, dry, comfortable sleeping quarters, together with massage of the affected parts and the application of hot packs, may relieve mild cases or assist in recovery.

In cases of posterior paralysis following distemper, and especially in cases in which the spinal cord has been severed or extensively damaged (as by an accident), treatment is usually of little or no value.

Urinary Calculi

The formation of calculi, or urinary stones, in the kidney is rare in small animals, but their occurrence in the bladder and urethra is common, especially in the dog.

Calculi vary in size, shape, and composition. In size they range from that of a grain of sand to that of a pea or larger. In shape they may be round and smooth or rough and irregular. They may consist of more or less hard concretions of salts, such as phosphates, oxalates, or urates, or of soft, waxy formations of nitrogenous material, when they are known as cystine stones.

The formation of the concretions (calculi) in the bladder may be due to a general systemic disturbance, to local inflammatory diseases of the urinary tract which produce an excess of salts in the urine, or to food or water rich in salts of various kinds.

The symptoms produced by bladder stones depend to some extent on their type, number, and size. Large, hard calculi produce the most pronounced symptoms. Urination may be difficult, and there may be small amounts of blood in the urine after severe straining, and constant dribbling of urine. Pus may also appear in the urine, there may be tenderness and pain in the region of the bladder, and the animal may move stiffly and stand with an arched back. In severe cases, general depression with loss of appetite and symptoms of uremic poisoning (chills, trembling, extreme weakness, and stupor) may develop.

Calculi in the urethra result from the stones that are formed in the bladder and lodge in the urethra. They are more common in the male than in the female dog. Affected animals make frequent attempts to urinate; there is evidence of pain and sometimes complete stoppage of urine, with a greatly distended bladder. Symptoms of calculi in the bladder may also be evident.

Treatment for urinary calculi is surgical.

Respiratory Affections

Inflammatory conditions of the different parts of the respiratory tract frequently occur in dogs and cats. The most common disorders are colds (inflammation of the mucous membrane of the nose and sinuses), laryngitis, bronchitis, pleurisy, and pneumonia.

Pleurisy and pneumonia may occur as complications in certain infectious diseases such as distemper in the dog, or they may be the direct result of injury, but for the most part inflammation of the different parts of the respiratory tract in pet animals is due principally to some type of direct infection. The inhalation of irritating substances such as dust and gases, sudden changes of temperature, exposure to rain and to cold damp winds, and cold damp sleeping quarters are all conducive to respiratory diseases.

In ordinary colds there is congestion of the mucous membranes of the nasal passages and head, with sneezing, coughing, and discharge from the eyes or nose.

An easily digested, nutritious diet, regular evacuation of the bowels and bladder, clean, dry, warm sleeping quarters, and the use of boric acid eye washes may materially assist in recovery from colds and other affections of the respiratory tract.

The treatment of serious respiratory diseases such as pneumonia and pleurisy, which are accompanied by symptoms of chilling, fever, difficult breathing, and weakness, should be under the supervision of a veterinarian.

Ranula (Salivary Cyst)

Ranula is a cystlike formation on the floor of the mouth under the side of the tongue. It usually appears in the form of an oval enlargement that may sometimes attain the size of a hen's egg. The condition is caused by an occlusion, or stopping up, of the salivary ducts. The affected animal has difficulty in controlling the movements of the tongue and in eating and drinking. Treatment is surgical. Temporary relief may be afforded by puncturing the cyst with a sterile, sharp instrument and forcing out the contents, but surgical removal of the cyst wall is necessary in most instances to effect a cure.

Warts (Papillomata)

Warts are small nodular growths occurring on the skin and mucous membranes in different parts of the body. They are of two types: Hard warts characterized by round, smooth, horny elevations, which occur especially on the eyelids, neck, head, and back of old cats and dogs; and soft warts characterized by a flat, rough, cauliflowerlike appearance, which occur principally in the mouth and on the genital organs of young dogs.

The appearance of large numbers of warts on dogs, especially in the mouth or on the genital organs in young animals, is not uncommon. The condition is considered to be contagious and is referred to as infectious buccal papillomata. Dogs affected with this type of wart should be isolated to prevent the spread of the disease to other animals. Buccal warts usually appear suddenly; they may persist for some time and disappear spontaneously without any treatment. Their presence in large numbers may interfere with eating and cause excessive salivation. In some cases applications of dilute vinegar to the warts will relieve the condition.

Intravenous administration of arsenical compounds is also of value in clearing up warts. Treatment for large warts is surgical and consists in their removal, followed by cauterization with silver nitrate.

Poisoning

Dogs and cats are poisoned mostly by accident, but occasionally they are deliberately fed poisoned material.

In a case of suspected poisoning, the animal should receive expert veterinary attention as soon as possible, since the immediate administration of specific antidotes, sedatives, and hypodermic injections to induce vomiting, as well as the use of the stomach pump and enemas for elimination of the poison from the digestive tract, is necessary to save its life.

In applying first-aid measures, an attempt should be made to remove the poison from the digestive tract by inducing vomiting (if it has not already occurred) through the administration of warm mustard water or salt water, and by the use of enemas or castor oil to produce bowel movements. Animals should be kept warm and the antidotes suggested below for each type of poisoning should be administered:

Arsenic and phosphorus poisoning occur mostly from eating food containing rat or insect poison.

In arsenic poisoning the symptoms are similar to those of gastroenteritis. There may be loss of appetite, intense thirst, signs of abdominal pain, vomiting, bloody diarrhoea, general depression, rapid shallow breathing, and complete collapse. Limewater, whites of raw eggs, or milk with raw white of egg may be given to allay intestinal irritation. A solution prepared from iron sulfate and magnesium oxide is the recognized antidote. Hypodermic injections of apomorphine are also beneficial in the early stages to induce vomiting.

Phosphorus poisoning usually develops slowly, sometimes requiring several days. The symptoms commonly observed are great restlessness, colicky pains, vomiting of material of a greenish-brown colour, swelling of the tongue, icterus (yellow discolouration of the visible mucous membranes), and general weakness.

For first-aid treatment administer 2 or 3 teaspoonfuls of milk of magnesia. Feed barley soup or oatmeal gruel, which may absorb some of the phosphorus. *Never give* castor oil or other purgative oils in phosphorus poisoning.

Recognized antidotes are copper sulfate, 1 part to 50 parts of water, or 0.1 per cent solution of potassium permanganate.

Lead poisoning in dogs or cats results from licking paints or drinking water or eating food from old paint cans. It occurs either in an acute form, characterized by acute gastroenteritis, colic, laboured breathing, trembling, general weakness, and coma, or in a chronic form from taking small quantities of the poison over a long period, characterized by bluish discolouration at the margin of the gums.

Strong solutions of coffee are beneficial as a stimulant. As an antidote, Epsom salts or Glauber salts, 2 teaspoonfuls to a glass of warm water, should be given. Raw white of egg and milk may also be given to allay intestinal irritation.

Strychnine poisoning in dogs is often caused by the administration of cathartic tablets containing small amounts of the drug and intended for human beings. An amount harmless to a man may produce poisoning in dogs because of their great susceptibility to strychnine.

Symptoms of strychnine poisoning, principally convulsions, develop rapidly, their severity depending largely on the quantity of the drug consumed. Spasmodic twitchings of the muscles of the limbs are first noted, followed by rigidity of the muscles and inability to stand. The eyes protrude, the jaw becomes locked, and the head and tail are drawn upwards. Death usually occurs after repeated convulsions. Prompt treatment is highly important and consists principally in the administration of a quick-acting emetic such as apomorphine given as a hypodermic to induce vomiting, and sedatives such as morphine, chloral, or ether to relieve spasms.

Phenol (carbolic acid) poisoning is usually caused by licking ointments or surgical dressings containing coal-tar products such as phenol, lysol, and creolin that have been applied to the skin. Cats are particularly susceptible to coal-tar products, and for this reason ointments, salves, and dusting powder containing them, should under no circumstances be used on cats. Neither should soaps containing coal-tar products, such as lysol, creosote, creolin, or tar and carbolic acid, be used in bathing cats.

The symptoms of carbolic acid poisoning are similar to those in lead poisoning. There may be the characteristic odour of phenol, abdominal pain with symptoms of colic, vomiting, excessive salivation, diarrhoea, difficult breathing, contraction of the pupils, and muscular trembling, followed by coma and death. Treatment consists in the administration of chalk and water or large doses of milk of magnesia as an antidote whites of eggs and milk are also of value. Aromatic spirits of ammonia or black coffee may be given as stimulants. A stomach pump may be employed to wash out the stomach.

Gas poisoning occasionally occurs through the inhalation of coal gas, carbon monoxide, or illuminating gas. The symptoms are difficult respiration, feeble pulse, bluish discolouration of the visible mucous membranes, convulsions, subnormal temperature, and coma, followed by death. Treatment includes placing the animal in fresh air, giving it aromatic spirits of ammonia to inhale, artificial respiration, and the administration of oxygen if it is available.

Food poisoning is observed mostly in dogs that run loose and obtain part or all of their food by foraging from garbage cans and refuse. The poisoning is produced by the consumption of rotten meat, garbage, or decayed carcasses. The symptoms may be similar to those of acute gastroenteritis, including vomiting, bloody diarrhoea, abdominal pain, and general weakness.

Treatment consists in removing irritant material from the stomach and intestines by the use of purgatives, the stomach pump, and enemas, and the administration of stimulants.

The danger of food poisoning as well as the risk of their acquiring infectious and parasitic diseases from contact with affected animals can be materially reduced by confining dogs and cats to their own premises.

Poison by snake bite–bites of rattlesnakes, copperheads, moccasins, and coral snakes–is not uncommon in farm and hunting dogs. The bite usually occurs on the face or legs and is shown by two tiny puncture wounds where the fangs have entered the tissues. A painful swelling quickly develops and spreads to adjacent tissues. There may be vomiting, convulsions, a weak pulse, and difficult breathing, followed by collapse and death.

Because of the rapid action of this type of poisoning, prompt attention is essential for successful treatment. If the bite is on a leg, a strong ligature should be applied to the leg between the bite and the heart to localize the poison. Small, deep incisions should be made into the wound and as much poisoned blood as possible expelled either by squeezing or by drawing it off with a small suction cup. The wound may be further treated by being washed out with a strong solution of potassium permanganate or pure hydrogen peroxide or by the application of silver nitrate.

Intravenous injection of polyvalent antivenin, a biological agent that has a specific action against several types of snake bite, is the most satisfactory treatment if given soon after the bite is received. When possible, dogs bitten by snakes should receive prompt veterinary attention.

Car Sickness

Car sickness is not uncommon in dogs, especially those with a nervous disposition. It is characterized by nausea when travelling in moving vehicles, the symptoms being drooling of saliva and vomiting.

This trouble can be prevented to some extent by withholding both food and water for an hour or more before starting the journey and also by giving the dog an opportunity to empty the bowels and bladder. The administration of 3 to 5 grains of sodium bromide before starting the journey and at intervals during a prolonged trip may assist in controlling vomiting.

First Aid

It is of the utmost importance that pet owners be informed as to what to do in the event of injuries, accidents, poisoning, and other emergencies. With such knowledge the owner can often take care of minor injuries and conserve the strength of the patient until veterinary assistance can be obtained.

Abrasions of the skin, cuts, and particularly bites are more or less common in dogs and cats. Such injuries should be washed with soap and warm water to remove all dirt and hair. It is important in bites or deep punctures to remove all contaminating material to prevent infection. The hair should be clipped from around the injured area and antiseptics such as tincture of iodine, tincture of metaphen, or mild antiseptic dusting powders applied. In areas where tetanus is known to exist, it is advisable to have a veterinarian administer tetanus antitoxin to animals receiving deep puncture wounds.

When excessive bleeding occurs as a result of severe injury, the hemorrhage may be controlled by the use of a pressure bandage (a wad of absorbent cotton applied to the wound and tightly wrapped with gauze bandage) or by a tourniquet applied above the wound.

In case of severe wounds, sprains, dislocations, or fractures, every effort should be made to limit movements of the injured animal to prevent further injuries to surrounding tissues, and professional help should be summoned immediately. The animal, which may be suffering excruciating pain, should be handled with extreme care so that it will not scratch or bite persons attempting to administer aid. When animals are transported for treatment to a veterinary hospital they should preferably be placed in a large well-padded box or basket.

Mild burns or scalds may be relieved by treatment with a 1-percent picric acid solution, by spraying with a freshly prepared 2½- to 5-percent tannic acid solution, or by applications of saturated sodium bicarbonate (baking soda). Later, mild ointments such as boric acid ointment may be applied. Severe burns over large areas of the body require professional treatment.

When pet animals are struck by automobiles or fall from a great height, serious internal injuries not apparent to the owner may occur. It is therefore advisable to have such animals examined by a veterinarian.

Since cats and dogs occasionally contract infectious diseases transmissible to man, such as rabies and ringworm, precautions should be observed in handling sick animals, or those showing abnormal symptoms. It is a good sanitary practice always to cleanse the hands thoroughly with soap and water after handling pets, especially those that show symptoms of being affected with some diseased condition. Scratches and bites inflicted by pets should also receive prompt and appropriate attention.

Spaying and Castration of Dogs and Cats

Spaying is a major surgical operation in which the ovaries are removed from female dogs and cats. The removal of the ovaries prevents sexual development and the occurrence of pregnancy. The periods of heat, or estrus, which are usually a source of great annoyance to the owners of female dogs and cats, are thus avoided.

The best time to spay the female dog is after the permanent teeth are cut and before the first period of heat, that is, between the ages of 6 and 8 months. In female kittens spaying should take place between the ages of 3 and 6 months. Spaying of old bitches and female cats is sometimes followed by apathy, laziness, and obesity.

Castration is a surgical operation for removal of the testicles in the male dog or cat. It is performed for the removal of diseased testicles, to curb extreme viciousness, to correct perverted sex habits, and to prevent wanderlust and interest in females. Castration is seldom performed on dogs but is a common operation in cats; castrated cats are sometimes referred to as altered or gelded cat. Cats of any age may be successfully castrated, but the best time to perform the operation is between the ages of 3 and 8 months. In some instances, castration has a tendency to increase the size of the matured animal, especially if it is performed while the animal is young.

Chapter 5

INTERNAL PARASITES OF DOGS AND CATS

Emmett W. Price & Paul D. Harwood[1]

[1] *Emmett W. Price is Assistant Chief and Paul D. Harwood was formerly Associate Parasitologist, Zoological Division, Bureau of Animal Industry.*

The life histories of the more important internal parasites of dogs and cats are here described, together with an account of the injuries they produce and the symptoms of infestation. The article closes with a rather detailed discussion of methods of prevention and medicinal treatment.

During the course of their evolution, dogs and cats have acquired an imposing number of different kinds of parasites–a total of more than 500. They include the Protozoa, helminths (worms), and arthropods. The arthropods, including fleas, lice, ticks, and mites, usually live on the exterior of the body; they are discussed in other articles. The Protozoa and helminths are all internal parasites, that is, they occur within the body of their hosts. Many of the internal parasites are of little importance, occurring so rarely as to be little more than zoological curiosities. A few, however, cause marked injury and even death to their hosts. Only the more important of the injurious species are discussed here. Measures for their control are given at the end of the article.

The damage inflicted by parasites on their hosts and the losses they occasion cannot be stated accurately, as no reliable statistics on these subjects are available. In the case of dogs, however, some idea of the losses that may result from parasitism can be obtained from recent estimates given by Judy (*16*).[2] According to these estimates about 900,000 puppies are whelped annually in the United States. About 30 per cent of this number fail to reach maturity. It may be assumed that about one-third of this loss–a conservative estimate–is due to parasites.

Parasites infecting adult animals do not cause spectacular losses as a rule, and often parasitism is not suspected until after the death of the animal. This is especially true of parasites occurring in the lungs and the circulatory and urinary systems. In fact, it is only during recent years that veterinarians have come to realize the injuries that can be caused by parasites other than the most common of those occurring in the intestinal tract.

The most widely distributed of the parasites of pet animals are those that have a direct life history, such as hookworms, large intestinal roundworms, and whipworms. Those that require intermediate hosts for their perpetuation, and hence have an indirect life history, are usually restricted to certain areas. The restriction is not absolute, however, since the heart worm, which until recent years was unknown except in the Southern States or in dogs that had at some time been in the South, has now become established in a number of sections of the country where suitable intermediate hosts are present. Other parasites, such as the dog eye worm, esophageal worm (infecting the esophagus, or gullet), and salmon-poisoning fluke, are definitely restricted in their distribution, even though the increasing traffic in dogs has offered many opportunities for them to become established elsewhere.

Protozoa

Only a few diseases of dogs and cats are caused by the minute primitive animals classed as Protozoa. Two such diseases are of importance in this country. One of these, canine piroplasmosis, has been known to exist in the United States during recent years only; it occurs in Florida and possibly in other Southern States. The other protozoan disease is coccidiosis. Coccidial infection is widespread, especially in dogs, but acute infections are either rare or are not generally recognized.

---

[2] Italic numbers in parentheses refer to Literature Cited.

Canine Piroplasmosis

The organism causing this disease is known as *Piroplasma canis.* It lives in the red blood cells and is somewhat similar in appearance to the organism causing tick fever (also a piroplasmosis) of cattle. As in the case of cattle, this parasite is transmitted from one dog to another by ticks. Several ticks have been shown to be capable of transmitting piroplasmosis, but in this country the most probable vector, or carrier, appears to be the brown dog tick, *Rhipicephalus sanguineus*, which is widely distributed throughout the South.

Canine piroplasmosis may assume either the acute or the chronic form. In the acute form of the disease the affected dog may show a rise in temperature, increased pulse and respiration rates, reddening of the visible mucous membranes, loss of appetite, and increased thirst. Jaundice is present in about half the animals affected. Acute cases are frequently fatal.

In the chronic form, fever may be noted during the first days of the infection, and in rare instances there may be an intermittent fever. The affected dog becomes listless, the mucous membranes are pale, the appetite diminishes, and the animal loses weight. Jaundice is usually absent, although it sometimes appears in the later stages of the disease.

In some respects the symptoms of canine piroplasmosis resemble those of distemper, and a positive diagnosis is therefore extremely important. Diagnosis is based on microscopic examination of the blood and the finding in the red blood cells of the causative organism of the disease. In chronic cases the organism may not be demonstrable, and it may be necessary to inoculate susceptible puppies with the blood from the sick animal in order to be certain that the disease in question is actually piroplasmosis. In inoculated puppies the piroplasms can be easily demonstrated in the blood in about 4 to 7 days.

Coccidiosis

Coccidiosis in dogs and cats is an intestinal disease caused by protozoan parasites of the genus *Isospora*. Several species occurring in dogs and cats have been described. Some infect the cells lining the small intestine, while others live in the tissue beneath this lining. The parasites multiply in these locations and ultimately give rise to resistant egglike forms, known as oocysts, which pass out in the animal's feces. These oocysts become infective in the course of a few days and serve to infect other dogs and cats. Dogs appear to be more susceptible to coccidiosis than cats, although coccidia are frequently detected in the feces of cats.

In light infections, no symptoms may be detected in either dogs or cats, but in heavy infections a diarrhoea, which may be severe and accompanied by the passage of blood and gas, appears at the time the oocysts are passing in the feces. Sometimes a slight rise in temperature may be noted. Under unfavourable conditions, as in heavy infections in very weak or young animals, death may result. Since coccidiosis may be confused with other intestinal disorders, a diagnosis must be based on the demonstration in the feces, by microscopic examination, of the oocyst stage of the parasite.

Flukes

Most trematodes, or flukes, of carnivores require two intermediate hosts in order to complete their life cycle. The first of these is invariably a snail, and the second is usually a fish, although in a few instances other animals may serve as second intermediate hosts. The most important trematode parasite of the dog is the so-called salmon-poisoning fluke, which is associated with a serious disease of dogs in the Pacific Northwest.

The Salmon-Poisoning Fluke

The fluke known scientifically as *Troglotrema salmincola* occurs in California, Oregon, Washington, and south-western Canada, where it is associated with a disease of dogs, foxes, and coyotes known as salmon poisoning. The parasites are very small, hardly visible to the unaided eye, and live deeply imbedded in the mucous membrane of the small intestine.

The life cycle of this fluke is complex. The eggs produced by the mature fluke pass out in the feces of the host animal and on getting into water develop embryos within 2½ to 3 months. The eggs then hatch and liberate ciliated, free-swimming larvae known as miracidia, which swim about and penetrate into a fresh-water snail (determined by investigators at the Oregon Agricultural Experiment Station to be *Goniobasis plicifera* var. *silicula*). After the miracidia penetrate into the snail they undergo certain changes and develop into small wormlike structures known as rediae. Within the body of the rediae are developed tadpolelike larvae known as cercariae.

When the cercariae escape from the rediae they pass out of the snail into the water. On coming in contact with fish belonging to the salmon family, the cercariae penetrate into the fish and become encysted (enclosed in protective structures) in the flesh and various organs. When infected fish are eaten by dogs or other suitable hosts the encysted parasites, called metacercariae, are liberated in the small intestine, where they develop into mature flukes in 5 to 10 days.

Salmon poisoning in many respects resembles canine distemper. The first symptoms following the eating of infected fish occur in 7 to 10 days, or about the time the flukes reach maturity. The onset of the disease is sudden and is accompanied by a temperature of 105° to 107° F. The animal is depressed, refuses to eat, shows increased thirst, and frequently has a discharge from the eyes. In many cases the face is swollen, causing the eyes to appear sunken. After 24 to 28 hours the temperature drops, and diarrhoea sets in, the feces at first being tinged with blood and later consisting almost entirely of blood. As the disease progresses, the animal becomes weak and emaciated; in about 6 to 8 days the temperature drops below normal, and death follows 1 to 2 days later. From 50 to 90 per cent of untreated animals die. Those that recover are not susceptible to subsequent infection.

Salmon poisoning has been shown to be a disease associated with fluke infection but not actually caused by the parasite. The causative agent of the disease appears to be a virus associated with the cellular elements of the blood.

A fluke, *Nanophyetus schikhobalowi*, which appears to be indistinguishable from that associated with salmon poisoning in dogs, has been reported in man in southeastern Siberia. No symptoms attributable to the presence of the parasite were observed, however.

Tapeworms

The tapeworms infecting dogs and cats in the United States may be roughly divided into two general groups, the armed forms and the unarmed forms. Species of both groups resemble each other in having a head, neck, and chain of segments. In the armed forms the head is provided with four suckers and a rostellum, or prominence, bearing two or more rows of hooks. The segments have one or two sets of genital organs, and the genital openings or pores are located on the lateral margins of the segments. In the unarmed species the head is provided with a pair of sucking grooves instead of suckers, the segments have only a single set of genital organs, and the genital pores are located on the ventral, or under, surface of each segment. A further difference between the armed and the unarmed tapeworms is that the armed species require only a single intermediate host for the development of the larval stages, whereas the unarmed forms require two intermediate hosts.

The Armed Tapeworms

For convenience of discussion the armed tapeworms may be sub-divided into the double-pored species, belonging to the genus *Dipylidium*, and the single-pored forms, represented by the genera *Taenia*, *Multiceps*, and *Echinococcus*.

The double-pored tapeworm that is of common occurrence in dogs, and cats in the United States is *Dipylidium caninum*. The adult tapeworm rarely exceeds 1 foot in length. The head is armed with 4 or 5 rows of tiny hooks, and the segments are shaped like cucumber seeds.

The single-pored tapeworms are, as a rule, much larger than the double-pored species. The head is armed with two rows of relatively large hooks, and the segments are more or less rectangular in shape (Fig. 1). The size of these tapeworms varies considerably. The smallest species, *Echinococcus granulosus*, is about one-fourth inch or less in length and consists of a head and only three segments. The other species may vary from 6 inches to 16 feet in length and consist of a head and numerous segments. The single-pored tapeworms are not so frequently encountered as the double-pored form and are more common in rural areas than in cities.

The life histories of the armed tapeworms are all similar in that, as already noted, only one intermediate host is required for the development of the infective larval stages.

The intermediate hosts of the double-pored tapeworm are usually, dog and cat fleas, and occasionally the biting dog louse. The infective larva of this tapeworm develops in the body cavity of the flea or louse and consists of little more than a head.

The infective larvae of the single-pored tapeworms develop in mammals, not in fleas or lice, and are usually referred to as bladder worms. The bladder worm consists of one or more tapeworm heads invaginated into a bladder, or vesicle, filled with fluid. Different

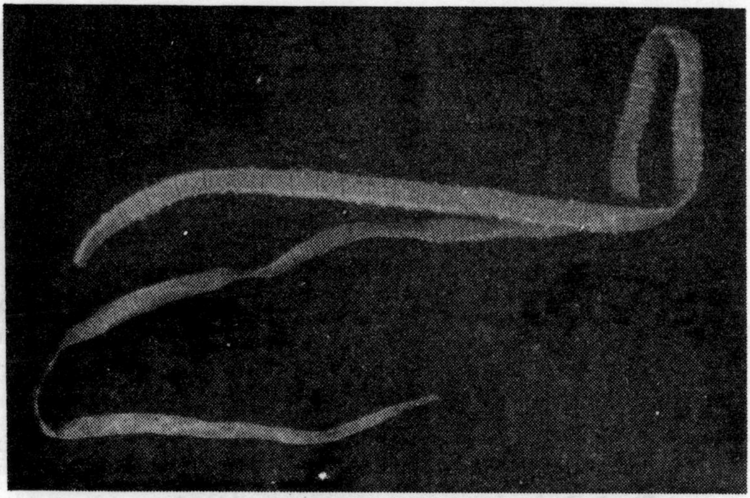

Fig. 1: *Taenia ovis*, one of the armed tapeworms of dogs. Natural size.

names are given to the bladder worms, depending on their appearance and the number of heads they contain, as follows: A larva consisting of a bladder containing a single head is called *Cysticercus;* when the bladder contains several heads it is *Coenurus* or *Multiceps* (Fig. 2); and when the larva consists of one or more bladders containing brood capsules composed of numerous heads it is *Echinococcus,* or a hydatid. When any of these larvae are eaten by the final host, the entire larva except the head is digested in the small intestine. The tapeworm head becomes attached to the gut wall, and in time, usually in about 2 months, a chain of segments is developed.

The names of the common single-pored tapeworms of dogs and cats, their intermediate hosts, and the locations of their larvae are given in Table 1.

The injury produced by the armed tapeworms in their respective hosts is not well understood. When only a few tapeworms are present, and even in some cases of heavy infection, no injury or symptoms may be detected. In some instances, however, there may be digestive disturbances, a disposition to vomit, general restlessness, and cramps. Nervous symptoms and skin eruptions have been

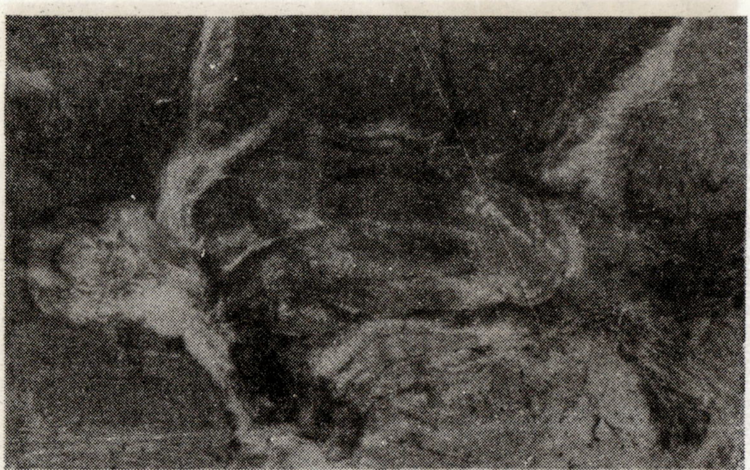

Fig. 2: Body of a squirrel, showing the bladder worm stage of *Multiceps serialis*.

attributed to tapeworm infections, but the connection between the presence of the parasites and such symptoms has not been well demonstrated. Tapeworm-infected dogs, especially house pets, are often a nuisance because the segments are frequently passed involuntarily by the animal and soil the floors, rugs, furniture, clothing, and bedding. Such detached segments are frequently referred to as pinworms; this is not a correct designation because dogs and cats do not harbour the true pinworms, which are a special kind of roundworms. The passage by dogs of a segment or a chain of segments through the anus often causes irritation, which is manifested by the animal's sitting down and dragging itself forward on its haunches.

Cats infected with the cat tapeworm, *Taenia taeniaeformis*, may show loss of appetite, transient diarrhoea followed by constipation, excessive salivation, and, occasionally, persistent vomiting. In kittens the abdomen may be distended, and the animals may exhibit evidence of acute abdominal pain.

Some of the armed tapeworms of dogs are of considerable importance as a cause of loss to the livestock industry, because of the presence of the larval stages in the muscles and other organs of

Table 1: The common single-pored tapeworms of dogs and cats, their hosts, larval name, and location in the intermediate host

Name of adult Tapeworm	*Hot of adult*	*Name of larval tapeworm*	*Usual intermediate host*	*Usual location of larva in intermediate host*
Taenia taeniaeformis	Cat	*Cystiercus fasciolaris*	Rats, mice, and other rodents	Liver
Taenia pisiformis	Dog, and, rarely, cat	*Cysticercus pisiformis*	Rabbits and hares	Omentum, mesentery, and liver
Taenia hydatigena	Dog	*Cysticercus tenuicollis*	Sheep, goats, cattle, snd swine	Omentum, mesentery, and lungs
Taenia ovis	Dog	*Cysticercus ovis*	Sheep and goats	Heart, diaphragm, and muscles
Multiceps multiceps	Dog	*Coenurus cerebralis* or Multiceps multiceps	Sheep	Brain
Multiceps serialis	Dog	*Coenurus* or *Multiceps serialis*	Rabbits and squirrels	Beneath skin and between muscles
Echinococcus granulosus	Dog	*Echinococcus granulosus*	Cattle, sheep, swine, and man	Liver and lungs

food animals. Some are also of importance as parasites of man. The double-pored tapeworm is sometimes encountered in human beings, especially children, and the hydatid stage of *Echinococcus granulosus* may also occur in man; a total of 391 cases of hydatid infection in man in the United States had been reported up to 1938.

The unarmed tapeworms of dogs and cats belong to the genus *Diphyllobothrium*, the best known species being the broad or fish tapeworm, *D. latum*. This species occurs in dogs and other carnivores in the Great Lakes region, where the parasite is endemic (that is, always present in the region) in man. A related species, *D. mansoni*, is of frequent occurrence in the West Indies and other tropical parts of the world. In some parts of Puerto Rico practically all cats and a high percentage of dogs are infected with this tapeworm. So far as is known, *D. mansoni* has not become established in continental United States. A third species of unarmed tapeworm, *D. mansonoides*, occurs in cats in New York and Louisiana, and has been found in dogs.

The life histories of these species are essentially the same. They require two intermediate hosts, the first of which are small crustaceans, or crayfishlike animals (*Cyclops* or *Diaptomus*); the second intermediate hosts may be fish, as in the case of *Diphyllobothrium latum*, or amphibians, reptiles, and mammals, as in the case of *D. mansoni* and *D. mansonoides*. In Puerto Rico the usual second intermediate host of *D. mansoni* is the common water frog, *Leptodactylus albilabris*, about 25 per cent of which in some areas are infected. Dogs and cats acquire these tapeworms by eating the second intermediate hosts containing the infective larvae.

Little is known of the effects on dogs and cats of infections with these tapeworms. Usually no symptoms of importance are noted, but symptoms similar to those caused by the armed tapeworms have been reported. Mueller (*18*) reports that infections with *Diphyllobothrium mansonoides* produce a marked effect on cats, stating that "Infected animals become emaciated, and the belly hangs down in a flabby condition. The coat is rough, with much shedding, and pronounced hunger and nervousness appear in hitherto gentle animals." This author writes further that "If the cat is promptly wormed on appearance of symptoms it makes a marked recovery. Animals which have been kept infected over long periods of time, however, are definitely stunted, and even after worming fail to regain weight."

Roundworms

The nematodes, or roundworms, are the most injurious of all the parasites of dogs and cats. Those species, such as hookworms and large roundworms, which do not require intermediate hosts, are the most injurious to young animals. They infect animals at an early age before any resistance to infection is acquired and may be responsible for the loss of entire litters. Such roundworms as heart worms and esophageal worms are usually found in mature dogs; these parasites require intermediate hosts for their development, and the time necessary for the larvae to become infective and for the worms to reach maturity is usually greater than in the species with direct life histories. Death seldom results from infection with worms requiring intermediate hosts, but the usefulness of the animals may be partly or entirely destroyed.

Hookworms

The hookworms are the most destructive of all the parasites of dogs and cats. Three species, *Ancylostoma caninum*, *A. braziliense*, and *Uncinaria stenocephala*, may be encountered. The first is the most widespread in its distribution and is accordingly the most important. *A. braziliense* occurs in the warmer parts of the world and is occasionally found in the South and Southwest. *U. stenocephala* is more northerly in its distribution; it occurs occasionally in dogs in the colder parts of the United States and in Canada, where it is a common parasite of foxes.

The hookworms (Fig. 3, *A*) are relatively small worms; the males rarely exceed half an inch in length, while the females are somewhat larger. The head end is curved upward and the mouth is provided with teeth or some other armature. The only certain way to distinguish between the different species is by microscopic examination of the head end. The mouth of the common dog and cat hookworm, *Ancylostoma caninum*; is provided with three pairs of large curved teeth; *Ancylostoma braziliense* has one pair of large and one pair of small teeth; and *Uncinaria stenocephala* has a cutting plate on each side of the mouth opening.

The life histories of the hookworms are relatively simple. The females produce numerous eggs, which pass out in the feces. In about 36 hours under favourable conditions a wormlike, active embryo has formed in the egg. In the course of 3 to 6 days the egg

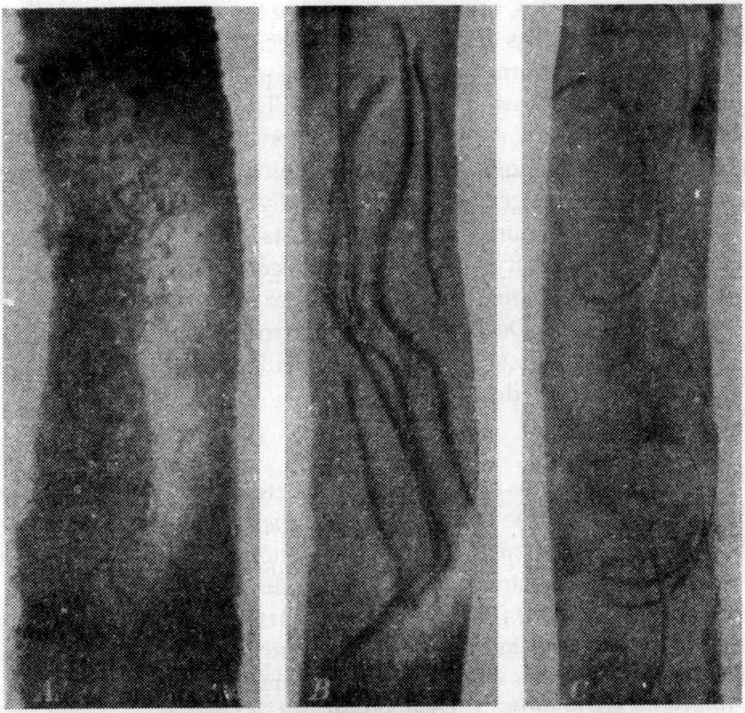

Fig. 3: Portions of the small intestines of dogs, showing infections with three of the common roundworms. *A*: The common hookworm, *Ancylostoma caninum*; *B & C*: the large roundworms, *Toxascaris leonina* and *Toxocara canis*.

hatches and liberates the first-stage larva. In about 3 more days this larva molts, or sheds its skin, and becomes what is known as a second-stage larva, which again molts in about 8 days to become the third-stage, or infective, larva. Infection of the host animal may take place either through the mouth or through the skin. When the larvae enter the host animal through the skin they get into the circulation and ultimately reach the lungs, are coughed up, swallowed, and finally reach the intestine, where they develop to maturity. When the larvae are swallowed with contaminated food and water they pass directly to the intestine. After reaching the intestine the larvae undergo two more molts and become mature, eggs appearing in the animal's feces in 3 to 6 weeks.

Eggs of the dog hookworm sometimes appear in the feces of puppies as soon as 13 days after birth, this early maturity being accounted for by the fact that infection took place before birth. This has been demonstrated to be possible in experiments conducted by Foster (*5*).

Hookworm infection in puppies and young dogs gives rise to a condition sometimes spoken of as kennel anemia. In the early stages of infection there may be digestive disturbances and diarrhoea in which the feces are streaked with blood. In severe infections the diarrhoea may be severe, and the feces may consist almost entirely of pure blood. A marked anemia, evidenced by the pale appearance of the mucous membranes of the mouth and eyelids, also occurs. Infected puppies rapidly lose weight, the eyes are sunken, and there may be marked symptoms of depression. Often no marked symptoms appear until 2 or 3 days before death.

The symptoms of hookworm infection are largely due to the irritation of the small intestine caused by the bites of the worms, to the removal of blood, and to the bleeding that follows the bites. Wells (*21*) has shown that a single hookworm may take as much as 360 cubic millimeters of blood a day and that 1,000 hookworms in the course of 24 hours could withdraw 360 cubic centimeter–an amount equivalent to about 12 fluid ounces, or three-fourths of a pint. The amount may actually be much greater, since in this calculation no allowance was made for blood lost by direct hemorrhage at the points of attachment of the worms. That the anemia from hookworm infection is due to loss of blood rather than to some toxin, or poison, secreted by the parasites is supported by the findings of Foster and Landsberg (*8*), which show that hookworm anemia is of the type associated with chronic hemorrhage.

The hookworm most commonly found in cats is of the same species as the common dog hookworm, *Ancylostoma caninum*, but it has been shown to be a strain especially adapted to live in cats and not readily transmissible to dogs. The symptoms produced by heavy hookworm infection in cats are similar to those in dogs. Because cats are usually house pets and have cleanlier habits than dogs, opportunities for acquiring heavy infections are not so great, and clinical hookworm disease in cats is rarely observed.

The larvae of *Ancylostoma braziliense* in the superficial layers of the skin have been shown to cause a type of dermatitis in man known as creeping eruption. The disease is characterized by a linear or tortuous eruption accompanied by intense itching.

Large Intestinal Roundworms

The ascarids, or large intestinal roundworms, are the largest of the worm, parasites occurring in the digestive tract of pet animals. These worms vary from about 1½ to 8½ inches in length, the males being considerable smaller than the females. On being passed by the host animal, the worms tend to coil in a springlike spiral, and apparently this is responsible for the name "spool worms" sometimes applied to them.

Two species of large roundworms, *Toxocara canis* and *Toxascaris leonina*, frequently parasitize dogs (Fig. 3, *B* and *C*). The former is more commonly encountered in pups and young dogs and the latter in mature animals. Cats, especially kittens, are frequently infected with *Toxocara cati*, but they may also harbour *Toxoscaris leonina*.

The life histories of the dog and cat ascarids are very similar to that of *Ascaris lumbricoides*, the large roundworm of man. Numerous eggs are deposited by the female worms in the intestinal tract of the host animals, and these are passed out in the feces. Under favourable conditions these eggs develop embryos in 2 to 6 days. The larvae undergo the first molt in the egg and the eggs then are infective. The infective eggs are swallowed by the host animal, and hatching takes place in the first part of the small intestine. The larvae of *Toxocara canis* and *T. cati* penetrate into the intestinal wall, enter the blood stream, by which they are carried to the liver and thence to the lungs, and finally are coughed up and swallowed. The larvae of *Toxoscaris leonina*, according to Wright (*23*), penetrate deeply into the intestinal mucous membrane, where they undergo considerable growth. After about 10 days they emerge and escape into the intestinal cavity, where they grow to fertile maturity.

Infection of pups before birth has been shown to be possible by Fulleborn (*9*) and by Shillinger and Cram (*19*). This accounts for the appearance of mature or nearly mature worms in very young animals.

The large roundworms are particularly injurious to pups and kittens. The commonest symptoms of roundworm infection are unthriftiness, digestive disturbances, and bloating. The hair coat is dead and lusterless, and the breath may have a peculiar sweetish odour. Large numbers of roundworms may cause obstruction of the intestine and even penetration of the intestinal wall. In heavy infections the worms may wander into the bile ducts, stomach, and even the lungs and upper respiratory passages. The occurrence of large numbers of larvae of *Toxocara canis* and *T. cati* in the lungs may cause pneumonia, especially in very young animals.

Whipworms

The dog whipworm, *Trichuris vulpis*, gets its name from its resemblance to a tiny whip. The front part of the worm is slender and hair-like, while the hind part is relatively thick. The total length of the worms rarely exceeds 3 inches, Whipworms are common parasites of dogs all over the world. They occur in the cecum, or blind gut, and sometimes, in extremely heavy infections, in the colon or large intestine.

The life history of the whipworm is direct, that is, no intermediate host is required for its development. The complete details of the life cycle are not well established. The eggs develop in much the same way as those of the large intestinal roundworms, except that the development of embryos requires from 2 weeks to several months, depending on temperature and moisture. When the infective eggs are swallowed by the dog, they hatch in the small intestine, and the larvae thus liberated ultimately reach the cecum, where they develop into mature worms. The time required for the worms to reach fertile maturity may be as long as 3 months.

The injury produced in dogs by the whipworm is not well understood. The worm attaches itself to the cecum by "sewing" its front end into the mucous membrane. In many instances these parasites appear to cause little damage, even in heavy infections. Occasionally the mucous membrane of the cecum may be considerably reddened and thickened, and this may cause considerable pain. A great variety of symptom of an indefinite sort have been ascribed to infections with this parasite, including digestive disturbances, diarrhoea, loss of weight, and general unthriftiness, as well as nervousness and convulsions. Though such symptoms may result from a number of conditions, the fact that marked improvement in an animal's health has in many cases followed surgical removal of the infected cecum lends support to the belief that whipworms are definitely injurious.

Heart Worms

The heart worm, *Dirofilaria immitis*, occurs most commonly in the dog but has been reported occasionally from cats and other hosts. The worms are slender and whitish in colour. The males are 5 to 7 inches in length and the females about twice this size. They usually occur in the right ventricle (Fig. 4) and in the pulmonary artery; in rare instances the adult worms may occur in other locations. This parasite is world-wide in distribution but occurs most frequently in warm climates. In the United States it is most abundant in the Southern States and those along the Atlantic seaboard as far north as New York. In most instances infection with this worm in dogs in the Northern States is traceable to the animals' having at some time been in the South, but in some northern localities the parasites have become definitely established.

The life history of the heart worm is complex. Instead of the females depositing eggs, as in the case of the hookworms, roundworms, and whipworms, active larvae are discharged directly into the blood stream. These larvae correspond to first-stage larvae of other nematodes and are, therefore, not infective for other dogs. The larvae are most abundant in the blood during the hours of darkness, but they may also be found during daylight. They continue to circulate in the blood stream until they are removed by some bloodsucking insect, such as a mosquito. Numerous mosquitoes belonging to the genera *Aedes*, *Culex*, and *Anopheles* have been shown to serve as satisfactory hosts for the development of heart worm larvae. These mosquitoes may not all be able to transmit heart worms, but the fact that the larvae can reach the infective stage in the insects, together with the fact that related worms are transmitted by mosquitoes makes them the most likely vectors. Fleas have also been regarded as possible intermediate hosts and this possibility has recently been strengthened by Brown and Sheldon (2), who found the infective stage of the heart worm in naturally infected fleas. While this observation is not conclusive, since experimental transmission of heart worms through the bites of fleas has not been demonstrated, it is extremely interesting and supports the contention of many dog owners and veterinarians that these insects may be important

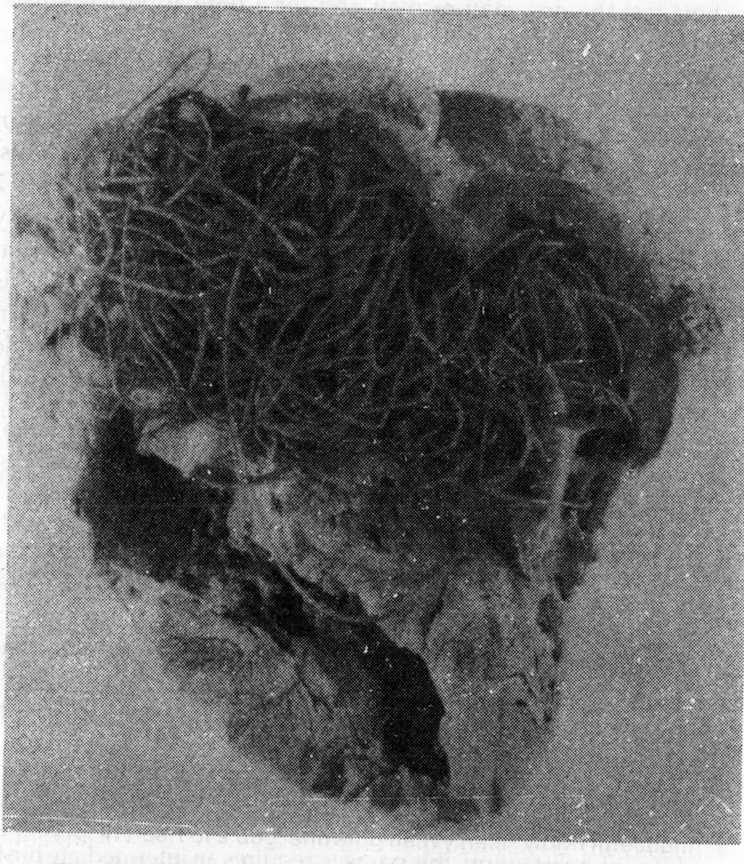

Fig. 4: Heart of a dog, showing heavy heart worm infection.

intermediate hosts. The time required for the development of the heart worm to maturity following the bite of an infected insect is not definitely known. Brown (*1*) has reported the finding of numerous larvae in the blood of an 8-month-old dog, which indicates that the worms reach maturity in less than 8 months.

The symptoms of heart worm disease in dogs may vary considerably, and in some instances no indication of infection may be detected until the blood has been examined. Usually, however, the first symptoms appear following vigorous exercise. The infected animal may tire easily, lie down, gasp for breath, and collapse. After a short rest the dog may recover and for a time appear normal. Coughing is also a common symptom. In cases of long standing, ascites, or abdominal dropsy, may develop and, because of poor circulation, the legs and other parts of the body may swell. Nervous symptoms, such as fixity of vision, fear of light, and convulsions have also been noted in infected animals.

The only way of making a definite diagnosis is by microscopic examination of the blood and the finding of active larvae. Finding larvae in the blood does not always indicate, however, that the adult parasites are present in the heart, since in many cases it has not been possible on post mortem examination to locate the worms in their customary habitat. This may mean that the worms responsible for the larvae are in some unusual location in the body or that they had died and become absorbed. The fact that larvae may persist in the blood after the parent worms have died is shown by the finding of Underwood and Harwood (*20*) that heart worm larvae could be detected in blood transfused from an infected dog into a non-infected animal for as long as 2½ years.

Esophageal Worms

The esophageal worm of dogs, *Spirocerca lupi*, is blood red in colour and about half the size of the large intestinal roundworms. Esophageal worms usually occur in tumors of the esophagus and stomach; as many as 30 individuals may be found in a single tumor. The species is distributed throughout the world; in the United States it occurs commonly in dogs in the Southern States.

Like the heart worm, this parasite requires an intermediate host for its larval development. When the eggs pass out of the host in the feces they already contain wormlike larvae. These eggs are eaten by dung beetles, in which they hatch, and the larvae penetrate into the body cavity of the beetles, where they become encysted. In about 2 months the larvae are infective for the final host. Should infected beetles be eaten by some animal other than the dog or a related host, the larvae re-encyst and remain infective. Such an animal is known as a transfer host. When the infective larvae are swallowed by a dog with either the beetle or the transfer host, the young worms are liberated in the dog's stomach and migrate to their final location. Many, if not all, of the larvae reach their final location after taking a circuitous route through the walls of the larger blood vessels, including the aorta. In the walls of these vessels, particularly in the aorta, the injuries produced by the wandering larvae result in degeneration of the tissues, with resulting scarring and thinning of the vessel walls. In some instances the injured aorta may become dilated, and deposits of lime salts may occur in the vessel wall.

The symptoms of esophageal worm infection depend on the location and size of the tumors. Tumors in the esophagus may cause constriction of that organ, resulting in difficult swallowing, vomiting, and loss of weight. Perforation of the tumors may occur, with the discharge of pus and eggs into the thoracic or abdominal cavities, and the infected animal may die from either pleurisy or peritonitis. If the tumors are located where they can press upon the windpipe or lung, coughing, difficult breathing, and suffocation may result. Sudden death may occasionally occur from rupture of the weakened aorta.

Lungworms

Lungworms are relatively rare in dogs and cats. Three kinds of lungworms are known to occur in this country, and in some districts the parasites may be of considerable importance. That little is known about them may be because they infect dogs and cats in rural areas, where the infections are not diagnosed.

One of the lungworms that infects dogs is known as *Filaroides osleri*. This parasite was first observed in Canada and has since been found in the United States. The worm is small and transparent and causes in the bronchial tubes wartlike tumors which may be sufficiently large and numerous to cause suffocation. Nothing is known of its life history or mode of transmission.

The cat lungworm, *Aelurostrongylus abstrusus*, is related to the dog lungworm and is common in some parts of the world. A few cases have been discovered in the United States, and the parasite is probably common in cats in rural districts. The worm is hairlike and occurs in the lung tissue. The females deposit their eggs in the air sacs, where they hatch, and the larvae thus liberated give rise to a pneumonia that may involve an entire lobe. According to Hobmaier and Hobmaier (*15*), the parasites require a snail intermediate host.

The capillarid lungworm, *Capillaria aerophila*, is related to the dog whipworm. It is primarily a parasite of foxes but also infects dogs and cats in fox-farming areas. The parasite is hairlike and whitish in colour and lives in the large and small bronchial tubes. So far as is known, the life history is direct, and infection occurs through swallowing infective eggs with the feed and water.

The presence of lungworms in dogs and cats gives rise to a more or less persistent cough. The animals also wheeze owing to the accumulation of mucus in the trachea and bronchi. Emaciation and general unthriftiness, together with wheezing and coughing, should be regarded as symptoms suggesting lungworm infection. Diagnosis can be made by microscopic examination of the feces and the finding of active larvae of *Filarioides* or *Aelurostrongylus* or of eggs of *Capillaria*.

The Kidney Worm

The so-called kidney worm, *Dioctophyma renale*, of dogs is the largest of the roundworms. It occurs in dogs and a number of other carnivores, especially mink, and has been reported in man on at least nine occasions. The fully mature parasite is blood red in colour. The females may attain a length of 3 feet and the thickness of the little finger; the males are rarely half as large as the females. The kidney worm is not a common parasite of dogs in the United States.

The life history and the mode of infection of dogs are not known.

The presence of this worm in the kidney causes pressure and destruction of the functional tissue. Only one kidney is affected, the other increasing in size to compensate for the additional work demanded of it. When the worms occur in the abdominal cavity, the commonest location, the eggs given off by the females cause a chronic peritonitis. The symptoms of kidney worm infection are not well known; dullness, incoordination of movement, and nervous symptoms have been reported in animals subsequently found to be infected. The infected dog may sometimes show evidence of abdominal pain and die suddenly following exertion. Diagnosis is impossible on the basis of symptoms alone, as symptoms similar to those reported may be associated with other conditions. If the parasite is in the kidney, a diagnosis is possible by finding the eggs of the worm in the urine on microscopic examination.

The Eye Worm

Only one species of eye worm, *Thelazia californiensis*, is known to occur in this country. This parasite has been described as occurring in dogs and has recently been reported in the cat, sheep, deer, and man. So far as is known, it occurs only in California. The worms are whitish and about half an inch long, and they live underneath the eyelids and in the tear ducts.

Nothing is known of the life history or mode of transmission. The parasite is related to Manson's eye worm of poultry, which is known to require an insect intermediate host.

The worms move about actively over the surface of the eyeball, causing considerable inflammation and a profuse flow of tears. Scarification (scratching) and ulceration of the eyeball may result from the activity of the worms, and opacity of the cornea and blindness may be the final outcome. In heavy infections the worms, may easily be found under the eyelids or crawling over the surface of the eye, but when the infection is light a careful search is necessary before a diagnosis is warranted.

Control of Parasitism in Dogs and Cats

General Measures

The control of parasites must obviously be based upon a knowledge of the organisms, their life cycles, and their resistance to physical and other factors inimical to their survival. Points that must be taken into consideration are the source of infection, whether the parasite requires one or more intermediate hosts, whether the route of infection is through the mouth or skin or by the bites of bloodsucking insects, the ability of the parasite in its infective stages to survive the action of sunlight and other natural physical agents, and the effect of chemicals and disinfectants on it during these stages.

The source of infection with parasites is for the most part contamination of the soil with feces or other excrements containing the eggs or infective stages of the organisms. Hence the most effective control measure is strict sanitation. In the case of such parasites as blood protozoans and filariids that are transmitted by insects, control consists in destroying the insects, protecting the host animals against their bites, or sterilizing the animal's blood by the use of medicinal agents. Where intermediate hosts become infected through eating infectious material passed by the definitive, or final, host, as in the case of tapeworms and some nematodes, control consists in strict sanitation and in preventing the final host from eating the infective stages of the parasite occurring in the intermediate host.

The general control measures discussed here are applicable to kennels and catteries where the animals are confined and where sanitation and other measures can be carried out. Under farm conditions and in suburban districts where dogs and cats are allowed to roam at large, such measures are difficult to apply, and the control of most parasites is largely a matter of treatment of the infected animals with anthelmintic drugs as discussed later.

Protozoan diseases–Piroplasmosis and coccidiosis require different control measures. Piroplasmosis is transmitted from one animal to another by ticks, and measures for the control of this disease must be directed toward eradicating the ticks in kennels and controlling them on the dog host; this problem is discussed elsewhere. The control of coccidiosis involves the same procedures as are recommended later for the control of certain of the roundworms, such as large roundworms and whipworms.

Flukes–Prevention of infection with trematodes, or flukes, involves keeping raw fish away from dogs and cats, as the infective stages of the majority of the fluke parasites of these animals occur in fish.

Tapeworms–The prevention of tapeworm infection may be summed up by saying: Do not permit dogs and cats to feed on infected intermediate host animals. Unfortunately, this recommendation is difficult to enforce when animals are allowed to roam at large and to have access to the carcasses of dead animals and to offal on the farm. House pets have little opportunity to become infected with tapeworms except the doubled-pored species, which is acquired through eating infected fleas and lice. Preventing infection with this tapeworm means controlling fleas and lice by destroying the breeding places of these insects and by the frequent use of insect powders and washes on flea- and louse-infested animals.

The armed tapeworms, such as *Taenia hydatigena*, *T. ovis*, *Multiceps multiceps*, and *Echinococcus granulosus*, are controlled to some extent through the enforcement of Federal and municipal meat-inspection regulations, which require condemnation and proper disposal of carcasses and offal of sheep, goats, cattle, and swine infected with larval tapeworms. The disposal by burning or burial of similar infected material on the farm should be practiced as a means of keeping dogs from becoming infected and later contaminating the fields and pastures with tapeworm eggs that may be picked up by livestock and develop into bladder worms.

Roundworms–The control of roundworms, with the exception of the heart worm, depends primarily on the prompt disposal of feces, keeping the animals in clean quarters and on clean ground, and using only clean utensils for feed and water. The runs or pens should be on clay and be free from sod. Clay soil is preferable to other types since it is more impervious than sand or loam, and parasite eggs and larvae remain on or near the surface where they are exposed to the destructive effects of sunlight and drying. Shady runways and pens should be avoided; such places are damp, and moisture favours the development and survival of worm eggs and larvae. Pens provided with wire-mesh floors that prevent the accumulation of manure are being used by some dog raisers with good results. The floors of such pens should be sufficiently high to permit the ground underneath to be cleaned readily.

There is no chemical treatment of value for destroying the eggs of such parasites as the large roundworms, whipworms, capillarid lung worms, and esophageal worms in contaminated soil. The eggs of these worms are provided with such impervious shells that disinfectants or other chemicals cannot penetrate them.

Hookworm-infected soil may be sterilized by the use of strong salt brine, a treatment that was first used in Canada for the control of hookworms in fox pens. This treatment was subsequently found to be effective for the destruction of the larvae of the dog hookworm in soil. The brine is prepared by stirring common salt into boiling water at the rate of 1½ pounds of salt to a gallon of water. The brine is sprinkled over the surface of the soil in an amount sufficient to saturate the earth to a depth of ½ to 1½ inches; about 1 pint of brine for each square foot of soil surface is necessary to accomplish this. The interval between treatments with the brine depends on the amount and frequency of the rainfall.

The prevention of heart worm infection is largely a matter of keeping dogs from being bitten by mosquitoes by confining them in mosquitoproof kennels during the late afternoon, night, and early morning. The possibility of transmission by fleas, which has already been mentioned, cannot be ignored, and kennels and dogs should be kept free from these insects. Destruction of stray dogs that may serve as reservoirs of infection and mosquito-destruction campaigns are measures that will tend to reduce the frequency of heart worm disease.

No control measures other than sanitation can be recommended for such parasites as the kidney worm, eye worm, and other worm parasites, the life histories of which are unknown.

Proper nutrition is an important factor in the prevention of losses from parasites. Foster and Cort (6, 7) have shown that hookworm-infected dogs kept on an adequate diet showed increased resistance and in some instances lost the greater part of their hookworm burden. When the same animals were put on an inadequate diet they again become susceptible to infection. Somewhat similar results were obtained by Wright (23), who showed that old dogs may be more easily parasitized by one of the large roundworms, *Toxocara canis*, if maintained on a diet deficient in vitamin A.

The Use of Medicinal Agents

In most instances the control measures already discussed, based as they are on a knowledge of the life cycles and other facts regarding the various parasites, serve to keep the parasites in check. They cannot be relied upon entirely to prevent losses from parasites, however, but must be supplemented, as occasion demands, by treatment of the individual animals with vermifuges and other agents.

Drugs and chemicals with specific action against disease-producing organisms, including parasites, have been developed largely during the present century. In the development of such agents the dog has played an important role by serving as a test animal, and as a result there are more specific treatments for the removal and control of the parasites of dogs than for those of any of the other domestic animals. Some of these treatments, notably those for the removal of the dog hookworms, are now commonly used for the removal of hookworms from man.

In spite of the many drugs of value for removing parasites from dogs and cats, there remain a number for which no satisfactory treatment has been discovered, such as those occurring in the respiratory and urinary organs, in the body cavities, and in tissues, such as the intestinal mucous membrane.

The advance of knowledge concerning the use of drugs in the control of parasites has led to considerable publicity regarding the value of such treatments. As a result, dog and cat owners have become "parasite conscious" and too often have felt that their pets should be dosed or wormed at regular intervals regardless of whether such treatments are necessary. Promiscuous dosing is a practice fraught with danger to the well-being of the animal. It should be remembered that all drugs for the destruction of parasites are poisonous to a certain degree and should be administered only when it is definitely known that the animal is suffering from parasitism. Diagnosis of parasitism is not always a simple matter. Many of the symptoms associated with parasitic infections also occur in connection with other diseases, and a laboratory examination may be necessary before a diagnosis of parasitism can be made. Consequently professional advice should be sought, and treatment for parasitism should be administered by or under the direction of a veterinarian. This is especially true in the case of cats, which require essentially the same treatment for a given parasite as do dogs but are much more sensitive to the toxic effects of drugs.

Protozoan diseases–Of the two protozoan diseases, piroplasmosis and coccidiosis, affecting dogs in this country, medicinal treatment is available in the case of the former only. Several drugs are known that are effective in varying degrees against the causative organisms in the blood. These treatments are administered as injections beneath the skin (subcutaneously) or into the blood stream (intravenously). The most recently developed and apparently the most effective of the treatments for piroplasmosis is acaprin, a synthetic drug known chemically by the rather formidable name of "N-N'-(bismethylchinolylium-methylsulfate–6–)urea." Like most drugs administered intravenously, it is toxic, and the dose must be calculated accurately on the basis of body weight. Clarvoe (3) recommends that appropriate doses be injected every day for 2 or 3 days, depending on the response. He states that if the animal has not suffered serious tissue changes as a result of the disease, recovery is usually prompt.

No specific drug is available for use in the treatment of coccidiosis. The indicated treatment for this disease is good care and nursing.

Flukes–The only disease of dogs in this country associated with fluke infestation that warrants medicinal treatment is salmon poisoning. This disease was formerly fatal to a large percentage of the animals affected. In 1938 sulfanilamide was found by Oregon investigators (*4*) to be a highly effective treatment. The drug was administered orally (by mouth) one to three times a day in doses of about 11 milligrams (0.7 gram) per pound of body weight.

Tapeworms–The several species of tapeworms occurring in dogs and cats are not all removable by the same treatment. The most effective drug for the removal of the armed species is arecoline hydrobromide, the use of which was first advocated by Lentz (*17*) in 1921. This drug is a drastic purgative and acts within a few minutes to a half hour or so after administration. The treatment should be given in the morning after the animal has fasted overnight, and food should be withheld for about 3 hours after dosing. The drug is not so effective against the double-pored tapeworm as against the other armed species, and it may be necessary to repeat the dose, since some of the heads may not be removed by the first treatment and regeneration of the tapeworm may occur in a few weeks.

Arecoline is not entirely satisfactory for the removal of the unarmed tapeworms, oleoresin of male fern being the most effective drug for use against these species. The drug should be given in appropriate doses after a fast of about 18 hours and should be followed by a purgative.

Both arecoline and oleoresin of male fern are toxic, and professional advice regarding the dosage, which must be computed carefully according to the kind of animal and its weight, should be sought before treatment with these drugs is attempted.

Large Roundworms and Hookworms–Since the most injurious parasites of dogs and cats are the roundworms that occur in the intestinal tract, investigations to develop satisfactory remedies for their removal have been extensive. Following preliminary investigations by Hall and Foster (*12*), during which critical tests were carried out to determine the efficacy of drugs previously reported to have anthelmintic value, oil of chenopodium and mixtures of oil of chenopodium and chloroform were found to have considerable value for the removal of large roundworms and hookworms from dogs. Owing to the moderate efficacy of these drugs for the removal of hookworms, further experiments were carried out with compounds closely related to chloroform. These experiments resulted in the discovery that carbon tetrachloride (*11*), a chemical widely used as a non-combustible cleaning agent, in doses of 0.3

cubic centimeter per kilogram (2.2 pounds) of body weight was highly effective for the removal of both dog hookworms and roundworms. This chemical was soon adopted by veterinarians as the standard treatment for the removal of these parasites. After making tests on himself, Hall suggested that carbon tetrachloride be given a trial as a remedy for the removal of hookworms from man. This suggestion ultimately led to successful experiments, and the drug was adopted by many public health officials as the best treatment for the removal of human hookworms.

Further tests carried out with other compounds resulted in the discovery by Hall and Shillinger (*13*) that tetrachlorethylene at the same dose rate was just as effective as the closely related carbon tetrachloride. Tetrachlorethylene soon supplanted carbon tetrachloride, as the latter drug was found under certain conditions to cause extensive and severe liver injury, and even death in some cases. Although tetrachlorethylene is much safer than carbon tetrachloride, it is less stable and, unless kept in a cool, dark place, may undergo a chemical change and become extremely toxic. Furthermore, in some animals it causes dizziness and even loss of consciousness. These effects, while quite alarming, are transitory, and the animal soon recovers if left undisturbed.

Later Wright and Schaffer (*24*) carried out extensive investigations of the halogenated hydrocarbons, the chemical group to which carbon tetrachloride and tetrachlorethylene belong, and showed that a number of compounds in this series possessed anthelmintic properties. Some were as effective for the removal of large roundworms and hookworms as tetrachlorethylene but were either too toxic or too expensive for general use. One of these compounds, normal butyl chloride, seemed to offer promise. Additional studies on this substance were undertaken (*14*) which showed that normal butyl chloride was as safe and effective as tetrachlorethylene. In addition to its effectiveness and safety, it did not appear to cause the alarming, though harmless, dizziness that often follows the administration of tetrachlorethylene. Normal butyl chloride is being tested extensively under practical conditions by veterinarians, and thus far encouraging results have been reported.

The amount of normal butyl chloride for dogs varies with the weight of the animal, and a schedule of suggested dosages is as follows:

Amount of drug	*Weight of dog (pounds)*
0.5 cc. (8 minims)	Less than 3
1 cc. (15 minims)	3 to 5
2 cc. (½ fluid dram)	5 to 10
3 cc. (¾ fluid dram)	10 to 20
4 cc. (1 fluid dram)	20 to 40
5 cc. (1¼ fluid drams)	More than 40

Whipworms–Until recently there has been no satisfactory treatment for the removal of whipworms. These parasites live in the cecum, or blind gut, which is situated at the junction of the small and large intestines. To be effective in removing whipworms, a drug must enter the cecum and come in direct contact with the worms; but the entry of a drug into this location is largely accidental, and in order to increase the chances of its happening, large doses of a drug essentially harmless to the animal must be used. Normal butyl chloride, which had been ascertained to meet this requirement, was administered in large doses to whipworm-infested dogs, with the result that an average of about 60 per cent of the whipworms present were removed (*14*). While this percentage of removal was not entirely satisfactory, it was greater than that attained by any other drug. The doses used were about four times greater than those effective for the removal of large roundworms and hookworms. The treatment may be repeated within a week if the results of the initial treatment prove unsatisfactory. Before treatment is undertaken the animal should be fasted for at least 18 hours; food may be allowed about an hour after dosing. Under ordinary conditions it is not necessary to administer a purge following treatment. If a heavy infestation of large roundworms is also present, a purgative dose of castor oil 1 hour after the administration of normal butyl chloride is recommended.

Another treatment for whipworms that appears to be promising was reported recently by Guthrie (*10*). It consisted of diphenylamine, in doses of 10 grams per animal, administered by mouth. This treatment removed 84 per cent of 537 whipworms from 5 dogs. Additional experiments to standardize the dose and to determine its safety must be carried out before the drug can be recommended for general use.

Intestinal worms in general–Whitney (22) has recently reported that hydrogen peroxide administered as an enema is very effective for the removal of all species of worm parasites commonly occurring in the intestinal tract of dogs. Since there is at present no single drug that will remove tapeworms, hookworms, large roundworms, and whipworms, this report is of interest. According to Whitney, a 1.5-percent solution of the drug is used. For dogs weighing 2 pounds a dose of 1½ ounces of the hydrogen peroxide solution was recommended, the amount being increased up to 24 ounces for dogs weighing 60 pounds. For successful treatment it is necessary that the animal vomit, and to facilitate this reaction a few ounces of the solution are administered by stomach tube just prior to the enema. This treatment should be used with caution, however, especially in animals suffering from diseases of the heart or other vital organs.

Heart worms–Treatment of heart worm disease is still somewhat of a problem. More or less satisfactory results have been obtained by the use of antimony compounds, but these treatments are toxic and expensive. Of the several antimony preparations reported to be of value against heart worms, the most generally used is fuadin, a compound known chemically as sodium-antimony-III-bis-pyrocatechin-disulfonate. Some dogs are peculiarly susceptible to antimony poisoning, and the treatment should not be attempted by the dog owner. Wright and Underwood (25) have shown, however, that the majority of animals can be treated successfully if the drug is administered carefully by a veterinarian. In appropriate doses it is administered either intramuscularly or intravenously daily over a period of 12 to 25 days, depending on the method used. There are a number of factors, such as the presence or absence of organic diseases of the heart, liver, and kidneys, the weight of the animal, and its tolerance for the drug, which must be considered before treatment is undertaken. If proper precautions are observed, about 90 per cent of heart worm cases can be cured after one or two courses of treatment with fuadin. It should be remembered, however, that a mortality of about 5 per cent may be expected even when the treatment is handled by competently trained individuals.

Literature Cited

(1) BROWN, HAROLD W. (1939). OBSERVATIONS ON THE DOG HEARTWORM, DIROFILARIA IMMITIS. North Amer. Vet. 20 (1): 49-54.

(2) _____and SHELDON, A.J. (1940). NATURAL INFECTION OF FLEAS WITH THE DOG HEARTWORM (DIROFILARIA IMMITIS). North Amer. Vet. 21: 230-231.

(3) CLARVOE, H.M. (1939). CANINE PIROPLASMOSIS. North Amer. Vet. 20 (7): 50-52, 53.

(4) COON, E.W., MYERS, F.C., PHELPS, T.R., and others. (1938). SULFANILAMIDE AS A TREATMENT FOR SALMON POISONING IN DOGS: North Amer. Vet. 19 (9): 57-59, illus.

(5) FOSTER, A.O. (1932). PRENATAL INFCTION WITH THE DOG HOOKWORM, ANCYLOSTOMA: CANINUM. Jour. Parasitol. 19: 112-118.

(6) _____and CORT, W.W. (1931). THE EFFECT OF DIET ON HOOKWORM INFESTATION IN DOGS. Science 73: 681-683.

(7) _____and CORT, W.W. (1932). THE RELATION OF DIET TO THE SUSCEPTIBILITY OF DOGS TO ANCYLOSTOMA CANINUM. Amer. Jour. Hyg. 16: 241-265, illus.

(8) _____and LANSBERG, J.W. (1934). THE NATURE AND CAUSE OF HOOKWORM ANEMIA. Amer. Jour. Hyg., 20: 259-290, illus.

(9) FULLEBORN, F. (1921). ASKARISINFEKTION DURCH VERZEHBEN EINGEKAPSELTER LARVEN UND UBER GELUNGENE INTRAUTERINE ASKARISINFEKTION. Arch. f. Schiffs u. Tropen Hyg. 25: 367-375, illus.

(10) GUTHRIE, JAMES E. (1940). PRELIMINARY OBSERVATIONS ON THE EFFICACY OF DIPHENYLAMINE FOR THE REMOVAL OF INTESTINAL NEMATODES FROM DOGS. Helminthol. Soc. Wash. Proc. 7: 84-85.

(11) HALL, MAURICE C. (1921). CARBON TETRACHLORIDE FOR THE REMOVAL OF PARASITIC WORMS, ESPECIALLY HOOKWORMS. Jour. Agr. Res. 21: 157-175.

(12) _____and FOSTER, WINTHROP D. (1918). EFFICACY OF SOME ANTHELMINTICS. Jour. Agr. Res. 12: 397-447.

(13) _____and SHILLINGER, JACOB E. (1925). TETRACHLORETHYLENE, A NEW ANTHELMINTIC FOR WORMS IN DOGS. North Amer. Vet. 6 (9): 41-52.

(14) HARWOOD, PAUL D., JERSTAD, A.C.., UNDERWOOD, PAUL C., and SCHAFFER, JACOB M. (1940). THE EFFICACY OF N-BUTYL CHLORIDE FOR THE REMOVAL OF INTESTINAL NEMATODES, ESPECIALLY WHIPWORMS, FROM DOGS. North Amer. Vet. 21: 35-41.

(15) HOBMAIER, M., and HOBMAIER, A. (1935). INTERMEDIATE HOSTS OF ALEUROSTRONGYLUS ABSTRUSUS OF THE CAT. Soc. Expt. Biol. & Med. Proc. 32: 1641-1647, illus.

(16) JUDY, W. (1940). DOG STATISTICS, SUMMARIES AND DIRECTORIES. Dog World 25(12): 6.

(17) LENTZ, WILLIAM J. (1921). TREATMENT FOR TAPEWORMS IN DOGS. Pa. Univ. School Vet. Med., Vet. Ext. Quart. 21 (34): 2-3.

(18) MUELLER, JUSTUS F. (1938). THE LIFE HISTORY OF DIPHYLLOBOTHRIUM MANSONOIDES MUELLER, 1935, AND SOME CONSIDERATIONS WITH REGARD TO SPARGANOSIS IN THE UNITED STATES. Amer. Jour. Trop. Med. 18: 41-66, illus.

(19) SHILLINGER, J.E., and CRAM, E.B. (1923). PARSITIC INFESTATION OF DOGS BEFORE BIRTH. Amer. Vet. Med. Assoc. Jour. 63: 200-203.

(20) UNDERWOOD, PAUL C., and HARWOOD, PAUL D. (1939). SURVIVAL AND LOCATION OF THE MICROFILARIAE OF DIROFILARIA IMMITIS IN THE DOG. Jour. Parasitol. 25: 23-33.

(21) WELLS, HERBERT S. (1931). AN OBSERVATION WHICH SUGGESTS AN EXPLANATION ANEMIA IN HOOKWORM DISEASE. Science 73: 16-17.

(22) WHITNEY, LEON F. (1939). HYDROGEN PEROXIDE AS A GENERAL ANTHELMINTIC FOR DOGS. Vet. Med. 34: 560-566, illus.

(23) WRIGHT, WILLARD HULL (1936). OBSERVATIONS ON THE LIFE HISTORY OF TOXOCARA CANIS AND TOXASCARIS LEONINA AND THE INFLUENCE OF ENVIRONMENTAL FACTORS ON THEIR DEVELOPMENT. Geo. Wash. Univ. Bul., Sum. Doctoral Theses 1934-36: 14-16.

(24) _____and SCHAFFER, JACOB M. (1932). CRITICAL ANTHELMINTIC TESTS OF CHLORINATED ALKYL HYDROCARBONS AND A CORRELATION BETWEEN THE ANTHELMINTIC EFFICACY, CHEMICAL STRUCTURE AND PHYSICAL PROPERTIES. Amer. Jour. Hyg. 16: 325-428, illus.

(25) _____and UNDERWOOD, PAUL C. (1934). FOUADIN IN THE TREATMENT OF INFESTATIONS WITH THE DOG HEARTWORM DIROFILARIA IMMITIS. Vet. Med. 29: 234-246, illus.

Chapter 6

MANGE OF DOGS

Emmett W. Price & F.C. Bishopp [1]

[1] *Emmett W. Price is Assistant Chief, Zoological Division, Bureau of Animal Industry, and F.C. Bishopp is Assistant Chief, Bureau of Entomology and Plant Quarantine.*

A dog suffering from a bad case of mange is a sorry sight, and the disease can easily have a fatal end. Three kinds of mites cause three kinds of mange; diagnosis is a job for experts, and cures are often difficult and may require long treatment. Here are the facts.

Mange is a contagious skin disease caused by microscopic organisms, known as mites, that are distant relatives of spiders and ticks. This disease, of which there are several types, affects a large variety of animals as well as human beings. It was probably known at least as long ago as the time of Moses, who stated that cattle and sheep that are "Blind, or broken, or maimed, or have a wen, or scurvy, or scabbed, ye shall not offer these unto the Lord, nor make an offering by fire of them upon the altar unto the Lord" (Leviticus 22 : 22). It seems reasonably certain that mange was one of the diseases referred to in this passage by the words "scurvy" and "scabbed."

The organisms that cause mange of dogs were not seen or described until the early part of the nineteenth century. The principal forms of the disease in dogs are sarcoptic mange, or scabies, ear mange, and demodectic, or red, mange. All three are relatively common and cause great suffering. If the sarcoptic or demodectic forms are allowed to go unchecked, they may soon reduce the most valuable dog to the level of a worthless mongrel. Early diagnosis and treatment of mange is important, and the dog owner should give prompt attention to any animal showing symptoms of the malady.

Sarcoptic Mange

Sarcoptic mange of the dog is caused by the mite *Sarcoptes scabiei canis.* The mites are very small, the largest specimens being little more than a hundredth of an inch long. They are approximately oval in outline, and the four pairs of legs are very short, the hindermost pairs not projecting beyond the margin of the body. The female mites burrow into the upper layers of the skin where each lays 20 to 40 eggs. The egg hatch in 3 to 7 days, liberating larvae that have three pairs of legs. The larvae grow by molting, or casting the skin, and after passing through a second, or nymph, stage become adult males and females, the entire life cycle requiring 2 to 3 weeks for completion. The larvae, nymphs, and males do not burrow into the skin, but live under crusts, or scabs, on the surface. The sarcoptic mite is not so prolific as some of its relatives, such as the ticks, but as the life cycle is very short, it has been estimated that a male and female may produce as many as 1,500,000 descendants in the course of 3 months.

Sarcoptic mange affects dogs of all ages and breeds. The disease usually makes its appearance on the head--on the bridge of the nose, around the eyes, or at the base of the ears. Sometimes, however, it is first noted on the front of the chest, on the lower abdomen, under the front legs, or on the inner surface of the thighs, and if it is not treated the entire body becomes involved.

Red points which soon develop into small blisters that are most easily seen on the unpigmented parts of the skin, such as the abdomen, are the first signs of the disease. As the female mites burrow into the skin, there is an exudation, or discharge, of serum, which dries and forms a scab. The affected parts of the skin soon become covered with branlike scales and later with grayish crusts. Itching is intense, especially in warm weather, or after exercise. As a result of the animal's scratching and of the irritation caused by the mites, the skin becomes thickened and wrinkled. The frequent rubbing and scratching favour secondary bacterial infections and the formation of sores. The hair may also become matted and fall out, leaving bare spots. Decomposition of the exuded serum gives rise to a peculiar mousy odour, which becomes more pronounced as the disease progresses. If the affection is allowed to go unchecked, the animal's digestion and other body functions become impaired, and death may follow in a few months. This form of mange is transmissible to human beings, and unnecessary handling of affected animals, especially by children, should be avoided.

Sarcoptic mange may be confused with other skin affections, such as demodectic (red) mange, ringworm, and eczemas of various sorts, and it is usually necessary to resort to a microscopic examination of scrapings from the diseased parts before a definite diagnosis can be made.

Ear Mange

Ear mange is caused by mites (*Otodectes cynotis*) which live in the external auditory canal. These mites are somewhat similar in appearance to those causing sarcoptic mange, but they are much larger and have longer legs. They may be seen with the unaided eye, either in the ear or in material removal from it, as minute, slow-moving, white objects. The life cycle of the ear mite is not completely known, but it is probably similar to that of the sarcoptic mite.

These mites do not burrow in the skin; they are found deep in the ear canal near the eardrum, where they puncture the delicate skin and feed on the tissue juices. Considerable irritation results from their presence, and the normal production of the ear secretions is interfered with. The ear canal becomes filled with inflammatory products and modified ear wax as well as mites, causing the dog to scratch and rub its ears and to shake its head to relieve the itching. Frequently the dog will hold its head to one side, and in severe infections it will run in a circle or show other evidences of nervous disturbance. The presence of the mites and the injuries they cause may favour bacterial infections resulting in inflammation of the middle ear and even of the brain.

Ear mange may be confused with inflammations of the ear due to other causes, and it is necessary that the diagnosis be confirmed by microscopic examination of material removed from the ear canal before treatment is instituted.

Demodectic (Red) Mange

Demodectic or red mange is the most common of the parasitic

skin diseases of dogs and also the most difficult to cure. It is caused by a wormlike mite, known as *Demodex canis*, which lives in the hair follicles and the sebaceous glands of the skin. The life cycle of this parasite is not well understood. The females lay eggs which hatch into young similar in appearance to the adults except that they are smaller and have only three pairs of legs. These larvae undergo molts as do other mites, acquire a fourth pair of legs, and become adult males and females. The time required for the completion of the cycle is unknown.

This type of mange may affect dogs of all ages but is most common in young animals, especially those of the short-haired breeds. The first evidence of demodectic mange is the appearance of areas from which the hair has fallen out. These spots are usually slightly reddened and commonly occur around the eyes, on the elbows, hocks, and toes, and elsewhere on the body. There is practically no itching at this time; itching may become pronounced as the disease progresses but is never so intense as in sarcoptic mange. In the course of time the hairless areas become larger and the skin has a copper colour, which accounts for the name "red mange" (Fig. 1); in severe cases the skin may appear lead gray or bluish. During this period the mites are multiplying in the hair follicles,

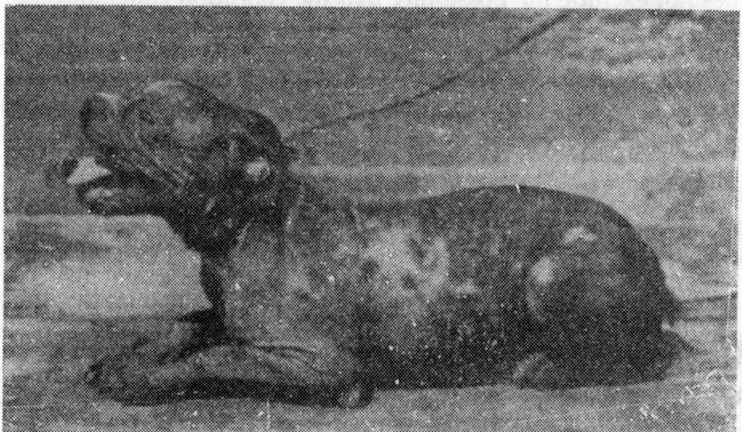

Fig. 1: A moderately severe case of demodectic, or red, mange. The hair has fallen out over the extensive light-coloured areas on the dog's body.

and inflammatory changes become evident, with the appearance of small pustules.

The hairless, or depilatory, type of demodectic mange, due to uncomplicated mite infestation, becomes complicated in the course of time through lowered resistance and the invasion of pus-producing bacteria which lead to the formation of small pimples, or pustules, in the hairless areas. As the pustular stage progresses the skin becomes thickened and is susceptible to injury by scratching, rubbing, or contact with various objects. There is very little itching in this stage of the disease. Poisons are formed by the bacteria in the pustules, and the absorption of this toxic material deranges the body functions and affects the general health of the animal, leading to emaciation, weakness, and the development of an unpleasant odour. The disease runs a slow course, often extending over a period of 2, years or longer. Unless it is treated, it usually terminates in death, although occasionally spontaneous recovery occurs, especially if the animal has been kept on a good, nourishing diet.

Demodectic mange may be confused with a number of other skin diseases, including sarcoptic mange, fungus infections, acne, and eczema. A definite diagnosis can be made only by microscopic examination of scrapings of the skin or of material from the pustules. Failure to find the mites, particularly in the early stages of the disease, does not exclude the possibility that the condition is demodectic mange, and it may be necessary to make several examinations at different times before arriving at a diagnosis.

Treatment of Mange

Medicinal treatment of mange, regardless of the type, should be undertaken only by or under the supervision of a veterinarian who is able to diagnose the condition accurately and to prescribe the proper treatment.

Ear mange is the type most amenable to treatment, since the mites are on the surface of the skin and are easily destroyed by the use of suitable insecticides. The affected animal should be restrained so that the ear canals can be cleaned and the wax and other material removed by forceps or a swab without injuring the eardrum. After being cleansed, the canal should be swabbed with one of the following mixtures: (1) 1 per cent phenol in glycerin, (2) 5 per cent phenol in castor oil or olive oil, or (3) a mixture of 1 part carbon tetrachloride and 3 parts of castor oil. An oil solution of rotenone is also reported to be effective. The treatment should be repeated daily until all traces of the infestation have disappeared.

An ointment consisting of 1 part by measure of derris powder containing 5 per cent rotenone in 10 parts of petrolatum or olive oil has also been found effective against the ear mange mites. The material is applied to the ears with a cotton swab. Usually two such treatments, 1 week apart, are sufficient to clear up an infestation.

Sarcoptic and demodectic mange are more difficult to treat since the mites in the skin are not easily reached with medication. Dogs affected with either of these types of mange should be clipped before treatment is attempted. The animal should be bathed and all crusts and scabs removed with the aid of a moderately stiff brush. In the most instances it is advisable to apply the indicated remedy to one-fourth of the body each day, so that in the course of 4 days the entire body has been covered. After a complete course of treatment the animal should be bathed and the same routine repeated until a cure has been effected.

In most of the effective treatments for sarcoptic mange the active ingredient is sulfur. One of the simple mixtures that frequently gives good results is an ointment prepared by thoroughly mixing 1 part of flowers of sulfur with 8 parts of lard. Another ointment that has given good results consists of 2 parts of sublimed sulfur, 1 part oil of tar, 1 part potassium carbonate, and 8 parts lard. Lime-sulfur dip as prepared for the treatment of scab in sheep is likewise an effective remedy.

Derris ointment similar to that recommended for the treatment of ear mange and a wash consisting of 4 ounces of derris powder (containing 5 per cent rotenone), 1 ounce of neutral soap, and 1 gallon of warm water have been found highly effective in curing sarcoptic mange. The wash should be well rubbed in with a brush. The surplus wash is taken up with a towel and the remainder of the material is permitted to dry on the animal. Two or three treatments are usually necessary to effect a cure. Exposure to sulfur dioxide gas has also been reported to give good results. The affected animal is placed in a gas-tight box from which his head protrudes, and the body is then exposed to the gas. Afterwards the head is treated with sulfur ointment. Cases have been cured after two or three such treatments.

The treatment of demodectic mange is often very discouraging because of the care, time, and expense involved. Many remedies have been used, but in spite of some cures there have been many failures. The most promising remedy appears to be a 1-percent solution of rotenone in alcohol or oil. The solution is prepared by dissolving the rotenone in a small amount of acetone and then adding the proper amount of either alcohol or a bland oil, depending on the kind of application desired; an oil solution is generally preferred because it tends to keep the skin soft and pliable. The remedy is applied daily, with a moderately rough massage, to the affected parts or the entire body, depending on the extent of the lesions. Constant treatment for several weeks is frequently necessary to effect a cure. The derris wash recommended for sarcoptic mange, applied every other day for 2 weeks then once a week for 4 weeks, has effected cures in a number of instances. Another remedy that has been recommended widely and has given good results in some cases consists in the use, once a week, of a preparation composed of 8 ounces of kerosene, 8 ounces of raw linseed oil, 1 ounce of carbolic acid, 1 ounce of oil of tar, and ¼ pound of sulfur. This mixture is applied with mild rubbing, but in using it not more than one-fourth of the dog's body should be treated at a time, as there is some danger of carbolic acid poisoning. Two or three complete treatments are usually necessary to effect a cure. With all these treatments, care should be taken, to keep the material out of the animal's eyes, as severe inflammation and even blindness may result.

In connection with medicinal treatment for either sarcoptic or demodectic mange, supplementary measures in the form of good, nourishing food containing adequate vitamins and minerals, laxatives, and warm comfortable quarters will enhance the animal's chances of recovery.

It should be remembered that the premises frequented by mangy dogs are infected, and disinfection is therefore necessary to prevent reinfection of the treated animals or the spread of the disease to healthy dogs. So far as possible all litter and bedding should be burned and the kennels disinfected with a hot, strong coal-tar-creosote solution. Where effective disinfection is impossible or impractical, as in the case of yards and large runways, dogs should be kept off such premises for at least 3 weeks to allow sufficient time for any mange mites that might be present to die.

Chapter 7

TICKS AFFECTING DOGS

F.C. Bishopp & Carroll N. Smith [1]

[1] *F.C. Bishopp is Assistant Chief and Carroll N. Smith is Assistant Entomologist, Bureau of Eutomology and Plant Quarantine.*

Not everyone realizes that the so-called wood tick is also a dog tick and that there are eight species of these creatures, several of which carry such diseases as Rocky Mountain spotted fever and tularemia. Few dog owners have not at one time or another had to deal with the tick problem. The most effective methods are described in this article.

As the terms "dog ticks" and "wood ticks" are commonly used, they refer to eight different species of ticks so similar in appearance and habits that few persons not entomologists are able to differentiate between them. All are of importance as parasites of dogs, and many will also feed on other domestic animals and human beings. Some of them serve as carriers of diseases of animals or man, in addition to inflicting irritating bites.

All ticks have somewhat similar habits in that they must feed on blood in order to reproduce. The eggs are always deposited on the ground or elsewhere after the female has become engorged with blood and dropped from the dog or other animal upon which she has fed. Among the different kinds of ticks, however, there are minor differences in life history, the hosts attacked, and egg laying and other habits, and also in the role the ticks play in disease transmission (*1, 5, 6, 9*).[2]

---

[2] Italic numbers in parentheses refer to Literature cited.

The American dog tick (*Dermacentore variabilis*), the most widely distributed and abundant species, is most numerous along the Atlantic and Gulf coasts, in the Mississippi Valley, and along the Pacific coast as far north as Oregon. Scattered infestations may be found in nearly all the other parts of the United States except the Rocky Mountain region and the Pacific Northwest. A closely related species, called the Rocky Mountain spotted fever tick (*Dermacentor andersoni*), occurs in the Rocky Mountain region, and a second closely related species, the Pacific coast tick (*Dermacentor occidentalis*) occurs in California and southern Oregon. The brown dog tick (*Rhipicephalus sanguinius*), a species having somewhat different habits, causes permanent outdoor infestations only in Florida and Texas but infests houses and other heated buildings in many localities over the entire United States. The black-legged tick (*Ixodes ricinus scapularis*) occurs throughout the eastern part of the United States, and a closely related species, the California black-legged tick (*Ixodes ricinus californicus*), is found in the West. The Gulf coast tick (*Amblyomma maculatum*) is found in the States bordering the Gulf of Mexico and the Atlantic Ocean as far north as South Carolina. The lone star tick (*Amblyomma americanum*) occurs in the eastern part of the United States and as far west as Texas.

The American Dog Tick

In many localities the American dog tick (*3*)[3] is the most important pest of dogs. In heavily infested areas dogs that are allowed to run freely frequently pick up several hundred ticks each day, and this causes severe irritation, a bad disposition, and loss of condition. Although the authors have observed no cases of dogs having been killed by these severe infestations, animals are known to have been destroyed because of their weakened condition, ill temper, and suffering, and canine paralysis has been attributed to the attacks of these ticks. In resort areas considerable economic losses are sustained when visitors avoid certain localities because of the injury to their pets caused by these parasites and the fear of being bitten themselves.

---

[3] See also BISHOPP, F.C., and SMITH, CARROLL, N. COMBATING THE AMERICAN DOG TICK, CARRIER OF ROCKYMOUNTAIN SPOTTED FEVER IN THE CENTRAL AND EASTERN STATES. U.S. Bur. Ent. and Plant Quar. Cir. E-454, 5 pp., illus. 1938 (Processed).

A strong incentive to keep dogs free of the American dog tick is the fact that the bite of this species transmits the dreaded human diseases, Rocky Mountain spotted fever and rabbit fever (tularemia). These diseases do not occur in every locality where ticks are found, and in localities where they do occur only one in several hundred ticks is infected, so that most persons bitten suffer no ill effects; but when the tick happens to be infected, a bite has serious results.

The American dog tick and related species pass through four stages–the egg; the seed tick, or larva; the nymph; and the adult. The eggs are laid in a mass in protected places on the ground, particularly in thick clumps of grass. Each female lays only one such mass, which contains 3,000 to 6,000 eggs. The eggs hatch into tiny six-legged seed ticks, which attach themselves to meadow mice or other small rodents. In 2 to 12 days they fill themselves with blood, drop to the ground, and shed their skins, or molt. The tick that emerges from the old skin has eight legs and is called a nymph. The nymphs attach themselves to small rodents and become engorged with blood in 3 to 10 days (Fig. 1), after which they drop to the ground and molt, becoming adults. The adult males and females, shown in figure 2,

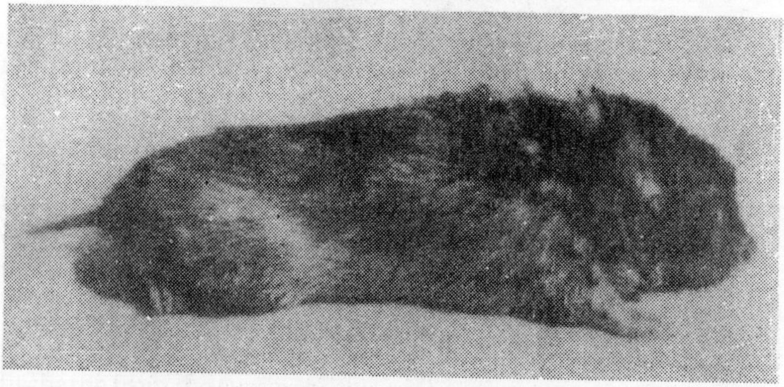

Fig. 1 : Nymphs of the American dog tick attached to a meadow mouse.

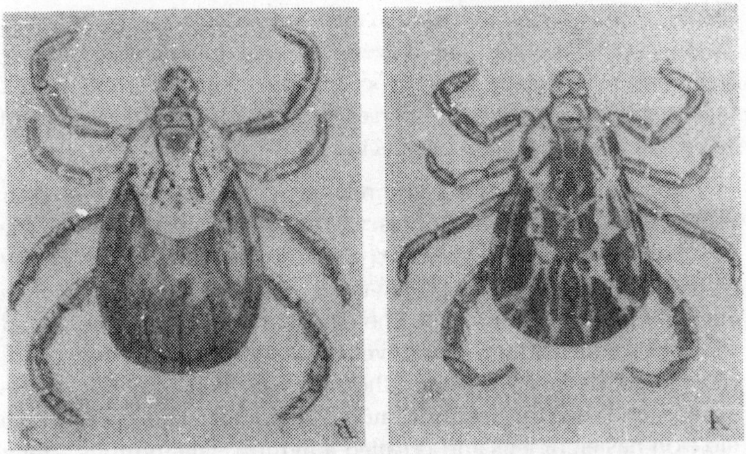

Fig. 2 : The American dog tick: *A*: Unfed male; *B*: Unfed female. Much enlarged.

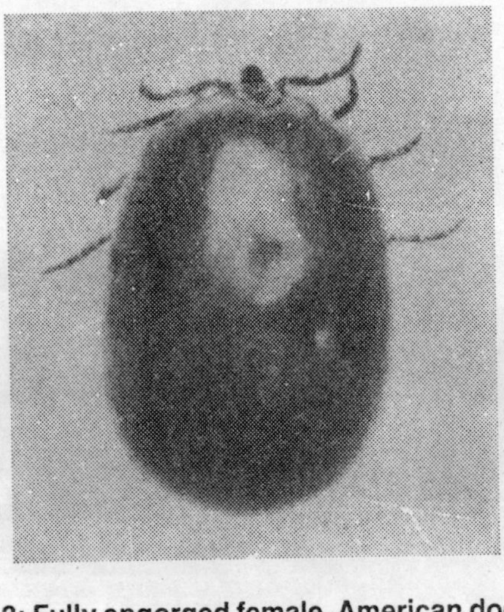

Fig. 3: Fully engorged female. American dog tick. Much enlarged.

also have eight legs but are distinguished from the younger stages by the white markings on a hardened part of the back called the shield. Adults of both sexes attach themselves to dogs or other large animals and feed on blood, but the females become tremendously enlarged, as shown in figure 3, while the males never increase in size. Mating occurs while the females are feeding, and when they have mated and become fully engorged, which requires from 5 to 13 days, they drop to the ground, lay their eggs (Fig. 4), and die. At no time do the ticks feed on anything but the blood of mammals. The larvae and nymphs may live for a year without feeding, and the adults for over 2 years. In the Northern States the adult ticks are most active in the spring and early summer, few being encountered after August 1, but in the South their activity is less sharply restricted by seasons.

The most effective way to prevent injury to dogs by ticks is to wash or immerse the dogs twice a week in derris dip. The dip is prepared by dissolving an ounce of mild soap in a gallon of warm water and stirring 2 ounces of fine derris or cube powder into the solution. These powders should contain at least 3 per cent of rotenone, the active insecticidal principle. If a suitable dipping vat

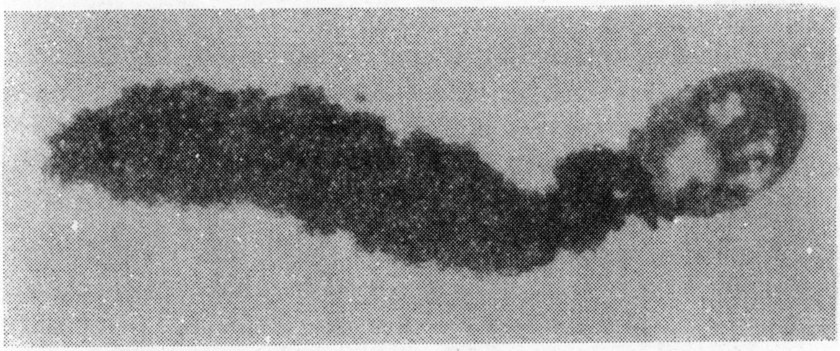

Fig. 4: Engorged female depositing eggs. Much enlarged.

is available, a large quantity may be prepared and used repeatedly, as the mixture will retain its strength for about 3 weeks if kept in the dark. If only a small quantity is prepared, it is best to place the dog in a tub and pour the dip slowly over it, working the liquid well into the hair with the fingers. The liquid may then be dipped up from the tub and poured over the dog repeatedly until the hair and skin over the entire body are thoroughly soaked. Care should be taken to prevent the dip from getting into the dog's eyes. If possible, the dip should be allowed to dry on the dog. The dip will kill the ticks that are attached, and for 2 or 3 days after a treatment the powder remaining in the hair will reduce the number of ticks that become attached and kill most of those that do. These materials act slowly, sometimes requiring as long as 24 hours to complete the kill. Occasional treatments will benefit the animals to some extent, but for good control the treatments should be given regularly twice a week.

If a dip cannot be used conveniently, derris or cube powder may be applied as a dust, care being taken that it penetrates the hair and reaches the skin. If the dogs breathe or swallow the derris they may vomit but will not be harmed, but it should not be permitted to get into the eyes. This treatment is also highly effective in controlling fleas.

Since the dog is the principal host on which the adult tick feeds and since each female lays several thousand eggs after feeding, treating the dogs regularly will not only bring them immediate relief but will definitely limit the reproduction of ticks.

When only a few ticks are present, they may be removed by hand. For this it is best to use tweezers or forceps, since human beings handling infected ticks may become infected with Rocky Mountain spotted fever. The ticks should be killed by being dropped into turpentine or kerosene as soon as they are picked off; if they are crushed, the blood should not be allowed to touch the skin. The hands should be thoroughly washed as soon as the job is done.

Methods of eradication applicable to all the different conditions under which the American dog tick exists have not been discovered but several things can be done to reduce their abundance, particularly around houses, in addition to the systematic care of dogs.

The destruction of rodents, particularly meadow mice, by trapping or poisoning, reduces the number of ticks in the following year by depriving the immature ticks of the hosts they require for larval and nymphal feeding (*10*). Almost complete eradication of the mice is necessary, however, if the reduction in the tick population is to be appreciable. Poisoning is more effective than trapping, but owing to the danger to other animals it should be carried on only under the direction of competent authorities.

Keeping underbrush, grass, and weeds closely cut tends to drive out rodents and removes protection favourable to the ticks themselves. Burning vegetation accomplishes the same results.

Close grazing of brushy and weedy areas by sheep will do much to reduce the tick population. If fine-wooled sheep are used, relatively few ticks become engorged on them, and many are killed by the wool grease.

Many of the ticks on an infested area may be killed by thoroughly applying a spray consisting of 1 part of nicotine sulfate (40 per cent nicotine), 1 part of soap, and 288 parts of water (this is about 8 teaspoonfuls of nicotine sulfate to 3 gallons of water). As ticks often concentrate on the sides of roads and paths, such places are most in need of treatment. Sprayed vegetation remains relatively free of ticks for about 3 days. More permanent results may be obtained by adding 4 ounces of sodium fluoride to the 3 gallons of spray, but this will cause some injury to the vegetation. Additional information on control is given by Bishopp and Smith in the circular cited in footnote 3.

The Rocky Mountain Spotted Fever Tick and the Pacific Coast Tick

The Rocky Mountain spotted fever tick and the Pacific coast tick are so similar to the American dog tick in appearance that they can be distinguished only by microscopic examination. They cause the same injury to dogs, but the Rocky Mountain spotted fever tick is particularly dangerous as a vector of the fever which gives it its name, as well as of tularemia and Colorado tick fever, and also as a cause of tick paralysis in dogs and human beings.

The life history and habits of these species are much like those described for the American dog tick, except that the larvae and nymphs feed on a much greater variety of mammals. Further information on the biology of the Pacific coast tick is given elsewhere by Hooker, Bishopp, and Wood (*6*), and the biology and control of the Rocky Mountain spotted fever tick have been discussed by several writers (4, 6, 7, 9).

The derris dip recommended for killing the American dog tick should be effective in destroying the Rocky Mountain spotted fever tick and others–except the ear tick–on dogs. Reducing the number of ticks on cattle and horses and destroying ground squirrels and other rodent hosts of the ticks have been advocated from time to time. These measures have not always been found to be practicable, but undoubtedly they do reduce the number of ticks. It is also worth while to clear away underbrush and keep dogs and livestock out of heavily infested areas.

Dog-Infesting Ticks Found in the Open

Other species of ticks that are found in the open and commonly infest dogs are the black-legged tick, the California black-legged tick, the lone star tick, the Gulf coast tick, and the ear tick. Their range has already been given. The Gulf coast tick resembles the American dog tick in appearance but can be distinguished from the latter with a magnifying glass. The lone star tick differs from others in having the shield marked with a single white spot at the back in the female and with two white semicircles at the back in the male. Neither variety of the black-legged tick has white markings on the shield, which is dark brown or nearly black.

The life histories of these species are similar to that of the American dog tick except that the larvae and nymphs feed on a greater variety of animals, including mammals, birds, and, in the case of the, black-legged tick, even reptiles. Also the larvae and nymphs as well as the adults of all but the Gulf coast tick feed readily on dogs. The Gulf coast tick in its immature stages feeds mainly on ground-inhabiting birds (2).

The treatment with derris dip recommended for the control of the American dog tick will also control the other species on dogs. Systematic treatment of the ears of livestock, especially on the inside, with commercial pine-tar oil will largely protect these animals and ultimately reduce the infestation on pastures. Clearing, burning, and grazing, as recommended, will assist in reducing the tick population.

Dogs are frequently infested by the spinose ear tick. This pest attaches itself deep in the convolutions of the ears and often causes irritation and pain, evidenced by the dog's scratching its ears, shaking its head, and holding the head to one side. Derris or cube powder (5 per cent rotenone) mixed with medicinal mineral oil (1 part of the former to 10 parts of the latter by measure) and dropped into the ears will kill these ticks. Only a few drops are required, but it is best to squeeze the base of the ear to work the material in among the ticks. A few drops of pine-tar oil (1 part) and cottonseed oil (3 parts) may also be used in the ears. Further information regarding this tick is given in Farmers' Bulletin 980. The Spinose Ear Tick (*8*).

The Brown Dog Tick

The brown dog tick is a particularly troublesome pest of dogs because of its habits. Whereas the other ticks of dogs require a vegetative cover and wild animal hosts to complete their development, the brown dog tick is adapted to life in the drier environment of kennels, houses, etc., with the dog as the only necessary host. It is also of some importance as a vector of canine piroplasmosis, although this disease is not widespread in the United States. Additional information on this pest has been published by Bishopp.[4]

The brown dog tick often infests houses in considerable numbers, both immature and adult ticks hiding around baseboards, window casings, and furniture, and in the folds of curtains. Dogs kept in houses are thus constantly exposed to attack and frequently become infested with hundreds of larvae, nymphs, and adults. As noted in the paragraph on distribution, this species has become established in many northern localities because of its ability to live in heated buildings.

Aside from the difference in environment and the fact that the ticks in all stages feed on dogs, the life history of the brown dog tick is like that of the American dog tick. The adults, however, do not bite human beings. This tick differs from the American dog tick in appearance in that the adult has no white markings on the shield, which is plain brown.

In combating the brown dog tick it is necessary to treat not only the infested animals but also their sleeping places.

---

[4] BISHOPP, F.C. THE BROWN DOG TICK, WITH SUGGESTIONS FOR ITS CONTROL. U.S. Bur. Ent. and Plant Quar. Cir. E-292, 3 pp., illus. 1939. (Revised). [Processed].

Clipping long-haired dogs aids in keeping them free of ticks but is not really necessary. Use of the derris dip according to the procedure recommended for controlling the American dog tick will kill the brown dog tick in all stages. As the dogs are constantly exposed to reinfestation, treatment should be given at 3-day intervals.

Infested dogs should be kept in one place, especially during their sleeping hours, to confine the ticks more or less and make the treatment easier. The kennels in which infested animals sleep should be thoroughly sprayed with undiluted creosote oil. This is the same material that is used for the prevention of decay in posts and timbers. Since it stains and is very caustic, it should not be used in houses or be allowed to come in contact with animals or plants. It penetrates wood and cracks and can be relied upon to destroy in a single treatment practically all the ticks in a building. If corrugated or other metal kennels or cages are being used, it is probably best not to use the creosote oil but to spray with creosote dip. The strength should be triple that usually recommended for disinfecting purposes.

The face and hands of spray operators, or persons applying creosote in any manner, should be protected, as creosote in this form is highiy irritating.

The use of a gasoline torch or "prickly pear burner" in concrete or other fireproof buildings destroys the ticks in the cracks and floors, but it is not approved. The use of a torch in a wooden building should be prohibited.

In dog and cat hospitals special attention should be given to having the cages and building constructed so as to reduce the number of hiding places for ticks to a minimum. Smooth concrete floors and walls are desirable, and cages made of metal give much less opportunity for ticks to hide than those made of wood.

When residences become infested, it is best to keep the dogs out of doors except when they are allowed to enter the house to serve as traps for free ticks. The baseboards, window casings, and other infested places should be sprayed frequently with one of the standard fly sprays, which are essentially kerosene extracts of pyrethrum. The ticks are quite resistant to sprays of this kind and must be wetted thoroughly if they are to be killed. In addition to the spray, the use of fresh pyrethrum or derris powder scattered behind baseboards and other hiding places is advised. If the dog is kept indoors it should be treated regularly as described. The treatment of the dog and the premises must be persisted in for several months to eradicate the pests completely.

Fumigation of infested houses is seldom advisable because the ticks are usually present in entryways, around porches, and in outbuildings where they cannot be reached with a fumigant, and they are also very resistant to fumigants.

Literature Cited

(1) BISHOPP, F.C. (1935). TICKS AND THE ROLE THEY PLAY IN THE TRANSMISSION OF DISEASES. Smithsn. Inst. Ann. Rpt. 1933, pp. 389-406, illus.

(2) _____and HIXSON, HOMER (1936). BIOLOGY AND ECONOMIC IMPORTANCE OF THE GULF COAST TICK. Jour. Econ. Ent. 29: 1068-1076, illus.

(3) _____and SMITH, CARROLL N. (1938). THE AMERICAN DOG TICK, EASTERN CARRIER OF ROCKY MOUNTAIN SPOTTED FEVER. U.S. Dept. Agr. Cir. 478, 26 pp., illus.

(4) COOLEY, R.A. (1932). THE ROCKY MOUNTAIN WOOD TICK. Mont. Agr. Expt. Sta. But. 268, 58 pp., illus.

(5) HERMS, WILLIAM B. (1939). MEDICAL ENTOMOLOOY WITH SPECIAL REFERENCE TO THE HEALTH AND WELL-BEING OF MAN AND ANIMALS. Ed. 3, 582 pp., illus. New York.

(6) HOOKER, W.A., BISHOPP, F.C. and WOOD, H.P. (1912). THE LIFE HISTORY AND BIONOMICS OF SOME NORTH AMERICAN TICKS. U.S. Bur. Ent. Bul. 106, 239 pp., illus.

(7) HUNTER, W.D., and BISHOPP, F.C. (1911). THE ROCKY MOUNTAIN SPOTTED FEVER TICK. U.S. Bur. Ent. Bul. 105, 47 pp., illus.

(8) IMES, MARION. (1918). THE SPINOSE EAR TICK. U.S. Dept. Agr. Farmers' Bul. 980, 8 pp., illus.

(9) PARKER, R.R., PHILIP, CORNELIUS B., DAVIS, GORDON E., and COOLEY, R.A. (1937). TICKS OF THE UNITED STATES IN RELATION TO DISEASE IN MAN. Jour. Econ. Ent. 30: 51-69.

(10) SILVER, JAMES (1930). MOUSE CONTROL IN FIELD AND ORCHARD. U.S. Dept. Agr. Farmers' Bul. 1397, 14 pp., illus. (Revised.)

Chapter 8

FLEAS

F.C. Bishopp [1]

[1] *F.C. Bishopp is Assistant Chief, Bureau of Entomology and Plant Quarantine.*

Fleas do so much harm and they are so great an annoyance to animals and human beings that it is worth while to maintain a perpetual campaign against them. The control measures outlined here are not difficult but require persistence.

Dogs and cats are all too often beset by hundreds of bloodthirsty fleas. Frequently these pests do pot confine their attacks to pet animals but overrun homes, barns, and poultry houses, sorely annoying human beings, livestock, and poultry.

There are many kinds of fleas, but those most important so far as the health and comfort of pet animals are concerned are the species commonly known as the human flea (*Pulex irritans*), the dog flea (*Ctenocephalides canis*), and the cat flea (*Ctenocephalides felis*) (Fig. 1). When the latter two species appear as troublesome pests in farm or city houses, they are always associated with dogs or cats. The human flea may breed on these animals and also on hogs as well as on man.

The sticktight flea (*Echidnophaga gallinacea*) is another species that attacks dogs and cats. The edges of the ears of these animals often become rimmed with hundreds of the pests, and they attach themselves in considerable numbers to other parts of the body.

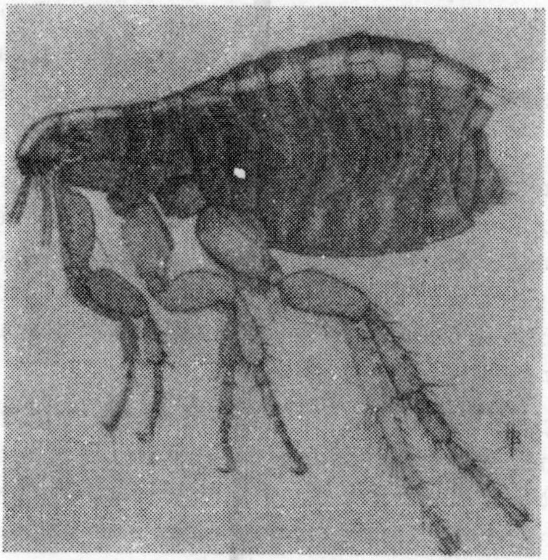

Fig. 1: A female cat flea. Greatly enlarged.

Needless to say, fleas are extremely annoying to dogs and cats, causing them to almost continuously scratch and bite in an effort to get rid of the pests. The coats of pet animals are soiled and roughened by the fleas and the scratching they induced. Fleas also appear to be connected in some way with summer eczema of dogs; at least, this diseased condition of the skin usually clears up when the fleas are eliminated.

The cat flea, dog flea, and human flea all serve as hosts for young stages of the dog tapeworm. The fleas swallow the tapeworm eggs that get into the dog's hair from segments of tapeworms passed by dogs. The eggs hatch and go through certain developmental stages in the fleas, and if one of the insects is then swallowed by the dog in biting itself--or accidentally by a child, as occasionally happens–the young tapeworm, in what is called the cysticercoid stage, passes to the intestine of the new host, where the worm attaches itself and develops.

All three of the species of fleas mentioned are also capable of carrying the deadly disease of human beings and rats, bubonic plague. At present, however, this disease occurs only in restricted areas in the West, and it is ordinarily transmitted by rodent fleas.

From the standpoint of human comfort and welfare, the most important aspect of the problem is the frequency with which homes become overrun by fleas that breed on pet animals and in their sleeping places, so that life in the infested house is well-nigh impossible.

The human flea is most often found in troublesome numbers in the Mississippi Valley and in California, where it frequently infests houses, stores, warehouses, and barns. Barns in which hogs are permitted to sleep very often become heavily infested. Horses, mules, and cattle are much annoyed in such cases, and of course human beings suffer greatly from the flea bites.

The sticktight flea (Fig. 2) is a common pest in the Southern States. It is not only troublesome to dogs and cats but is a serious pest of poultry and a source of considerable annoyance to persons who tend the fowls. Young chickens and turkeys are sometimes

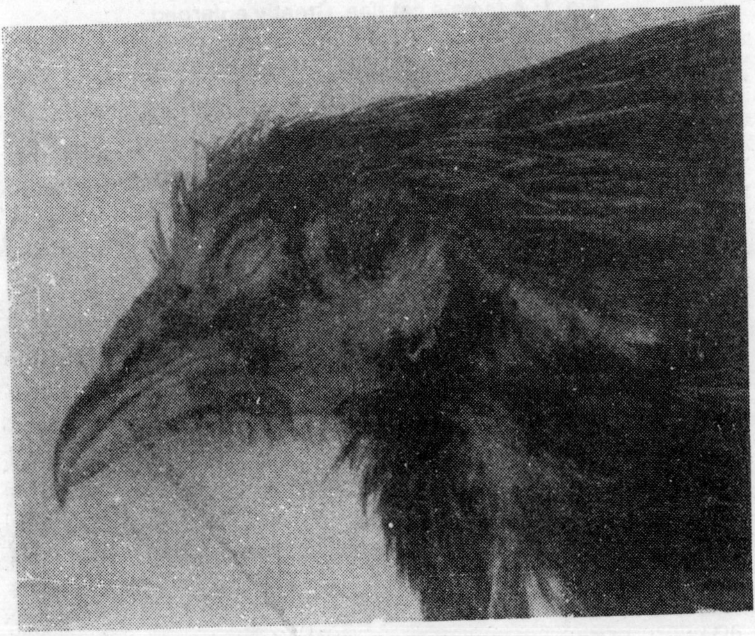

Fig. 2: Sticktight fleas on the head of a chicken.

killed by heavy infestations, grown fowls become weakened, and egg production is greatly reduced.

The ability of fleas to jump, bite, and elude one's best efforts to capture them is well known. Few people realize, however, that these pests must have warm-blooded animals on which to feed and that the young fleas, which resemble maggots, live and develop in the dust and debris in the sleeping places of animals. The oval white eggs are deposited while the fleas are on their hosts. The eggs then drop to the floor or ground and in few days hatch into minute maggotlike larvae which complete their growth in 2 weeks or more, depending on the temperature. The larva spins a cocoon about the size of a wheat kernel around itself, and in from 1 week to 2 or 3 months the adult flea emerges. Most of the life of the adult fleas is spent on animals. The attacks on human beings are mainly by newly emerged fleas that have not yet found an animal on which to live.

The attack on fleas must be directed against the adults on dogs, cats, and hogs, and against the immature stages of the fleas on the floor or ground.

Fleas on dogs and cats are easily destroyed by the application of a small amount of derris or cube powder scattered through the hair next to the skin along the neck and back of the animal (Fig.3). Fresh, finely ground pyrethrum powder dusted into the hair is also effective. Washing the animal in water containing derris or cube powder and soap is an excellent method of control. Two ounces of the powder and an ounce of neutral soap–preferably in flaked form-are mixed with a gallon of water. This is applied to the animal either by dipping or washing. The surplus water is removed with a towel and the remaining solution left on the animal.

Since fleas are continually picked up by dogs and cats that are allowed to run free, the treatment usually has to be repeated every 10 days or 2 weeks.

Fleas on hogs may be killed by sprinkling the backs of the animals lightly with crude petroleum or strained crankcase oil. Poultry need not be treated, because infestations of the sticktight flea can be wiped out by treating the breeding places as described in the following paragraph.

The destruction of the immature fleas on infested premises is accomplished by cleaning out and burning straw and other debris

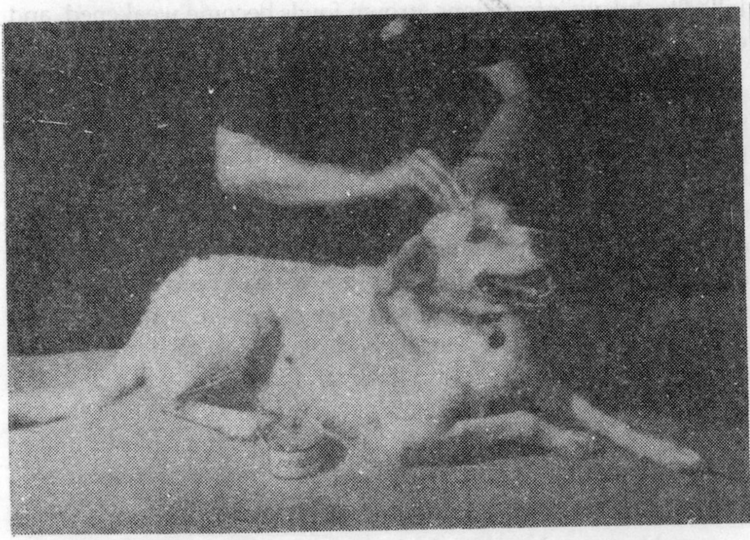

Fig. 3: A dog being dusted with derris powder for flea control.

from the sleeping places of the animals and spraying the ground thoroughly with creosote oil. This treatment also kills any adult fleas present. Creosote oil, commonly used as a wood preserver, is destructive to plants, stains paint, and is caustic to animals. Its use, therefore, is limited to outbuildings and basements where nothing subject to injury is stored. It should be applied with a good force pump, such as a bucket pump with a strong hose and secure connections. Creosote oil is reasonable in price so that it may be used freely on the ground and in and around barns where heavy infestations occur.

Fleas sometimes spread to lawns from heavily infested sheltered places, such as a garage and the ground beneath a porch. Keeping the grass closely cut will usually cause the fleas to die out in a short time. If they persist, spraying with nicotine sulfate at the rate of 6 teaspoonfuls to 1 gallon of warm soapy water will be effective.

In stores and in the living quarters in houses, creosote oil cannot be used. Flaked naphthalene is recommended for such situations, and it may also be used in basements. It should be scattered thickly over floors and infested furniture, after which the rooms should be vacated and left closed for 48 hours or longer. This kills both the adult and the young fleas. The naphthalene remaining after treatment may be swept up and saved in a tight container for future use.

If only an occasional flea is present in a house, fly spray may be used, but only the insects actually struck by the spray are killed.

There is little reason for pet animals to suffer from fleas and for people to be practically driven from their homes by these pests when simple, inexpensive, and effective weapons are at hand to use against them.

Chapter 9

RUNNING FITS (FRIGHT DISEASE)

C.D. Stein[1]

[1] *C.D. Stein is Veterinarian, Pathological Division, Bureau of Animal Industry.*

Fright disease is seldom fatal, but it can be very alarming to the dog owner who suddenly encounters it and confuses the condition with rabies. Here is a summary of the little that is known about this mysterious malady.

Running fits is a nervous affection of dogs commonly known also as fright disease, barking fits, furious fits, or canine hysteria.. The condition occurs in dogs of all breeds, of all ages, of both sexes, and at all times of the year. Although more or less prevalent throughout the United States, it seems to be more common in the Southern States than elsewhere.

Symptoms

The condition is characterized by periodic attacks of running and barking, together with manifestations of excitement and great fear. Between the attacks the animal usually appears normal, though sometimes becoming dull and listless. Usually the first symptoms noticed are restlessness, a staring expression of the eyes, and fright. In most instances the affected animal suddenly starts to run and bark as if pursued. The attacks, lasting from a few minutes to a half hour or longer, may occur at intervals of days, weeks, or months and may continue over a period of years. The mortality rate is usually low.

In mild attacks, after a short period of running, the dog will hide in a dark place, coming out later seemingly normal. Severe attacks may terminate in spasms or convulsions and may be accompanied by champing of the jaws, with a copious flow of saliva or involuntary passage of feces and urine. Less frequently the animal will remain timid or in a state of fear, will bark or snap at the slightest provocation, and will fail to recognize or obey commands given by its master. Occasionally the animal will suddenly commence to yelp and run until it falls exhausted. This type of attack occurs most frequently in hunting dogs.

The fits or convulsions that sometimes occur in young puppies heavily infested with intestinal parasites or cutting the permanent teeth should not be confused with this condition.

The symptoms of running fits are sometimes thought to be those of rabies because of the common but mistaken belief that a mad dog rushes wildly through the streets. Those who know the symptoms of rabies, however, seldom confound the two diseases. A veterinarian should be consulted when there is doubt as to the true nature of the trouble.

Theories as to Cause

The basic cause of running fits is still unknown. Several theories have been advanced, suggesting as the cause specific infection, hereditary predisposition, inbreeding, circulatory disturbances, faulty or deficient diet, indigestion, alimentary toxemias, foreign bodies in the digestive tract, parasitic infestation, estrum (heat), and sundry irritations and excitments. None of these theories, however, have been substantiated by sound experimental evidence.

Practicing veterinarians and investigators in the Bureau of Animal Industry and elsewhere have frequently observed that improper feeding, especially a long-continued diet composed largely of meal, cereals, breadstuffs, or dog biscuits, may produce a condition much like running fits, particularly in dogs that are kept confined. On the other hand, dogs that have liberty to run about and are on a diet in which meat plays a major part seldom develop the disease.

In recent years considerable attention have been given by investigators to dietary deficiency as a cause of running fits.[2] Walston[3] reported experimental evidence to indicate that the affection may be due to vitamin A deficiency. Dogs affected with this condition and fed largely on cereals recovered when the diet was changed so as to contain more vitamin A. Patton,[4] working with prepared dog foods processed by heat, reported experimental evidence to indicate that running fits may be a vitamin B_1 deficiency and advocated the administration of thiamin in treatment.

Arnold and Elvehjem[5] reported experiments in which symptoms of running fits in dogs were produced by foods that had been subjected to high temperatures. They suggest that the deficiency in heat-processed dog foods is in the protein rather than the vitamin content. Morgan[6] reported that heated proteins show a decrease in biological value, that vitamin B_1 withstands heat poorly and is likely to be low in all heat-treated dog foods, and that the food stuffs in all diets on which symptoms of running fits have been produced experimentally were baked or autoclaved (cooked by steam under pressure).

Schlotthauer,[7] on the other hand, reported that he was unable to produce symptoms of running fits in normal dogs by feeding heat-treated dog food or by various diets deficient in vitamin B_1. He suggests that running fits are produced in normal dogs by some toxic substance in the diet, but that they may be produced in dogs with, hereditary epileptic tendencies or in dogs infected with neurotropic organisms (those affecting the nerves) by feeding irritating substances or by deficient diets.

---

[2] For a further brief discussion of nutritional aspects of the disease.

[3] WALSTON, H.D. HYSTERIA IN DOGS. Nature [London] 132 (3328): 243. 1938.

[4] PATTON, JOHN W. FRIGHT DISEASE AN AVITAMINOSIS. Vet. Med. 34: 372-381, illus. 1939.

[5] ARNOLD, AARON, AND ELVEHJEM, C.A. IS RUNNING FITS A DEFICIENCY DISEASE? Amer. Vet. Med. Assoc. Jour. 95: 303-308. illus. 1939.

[6] MORGAN, AGNES FAY. DEFICIENCIES AND FALLACIES IN CANINE DIET. North Amer. Vet. 21: 476-483. 1940.

[7] SCHLOTTHAUER, CARL, F. FRIGHT DISEASE (RUNNING FITS) NOT A DIETARY DEFICIENCY.

Treatment and Prevention

In the treatment of this affection and in the prevention of further attacks, careful regulation of the diet of affected dogs is of first importance. Fresh meat, milk, and eggs should constitute a large part of the diet. The importance of fresh meat in the diet of a dog is stressed. The bowels must be well regulated at all times. Faulty sanitary conditions should be corrected, and care should be taken to prevent overexertion or undue excitement. At the present time no specific medicinal treatment is known.

Since infestation with parasites, constipation, indigestible material in the digestive tract, occlusion, or stoppage, of the anal pouches, or ear mites may aggravate mild affections of running fits and intensify the symptoms, measures for detecting and correcting any of these difficulties must also be included in the treatment.

In animals that do not have liberty to run about, the occasional use of small amounts of cod-liver oil, calcium lactate, and yeast as supplements is the regular diet is sometimes advisable.

During an attack, if affected animals are placed in a dark room, kept free from annoyance, and not molested, they will often recover in a short time. Following recovery, the animal should be kept as quiet as possible to avoid a recurrence of symptoms. Dogs that remain in a state of nervousness or show signs of increased nervous irritability should be given nerve sedatives. In some cases the removal of irritating indigestible material from the digestive tract by intestinal irrigation is followed by immediate improvement. It is suggested that actual treatment be undertaken by a qualified veterinarian only.

Chapter 10

NON-PARASITIC SKIN DISEASES OF DOGS AND CATS

C.D. Stein[1]

[1] *C.D. Stein is Veterinarian, Pathological Division, Bureau of Animal Industry.*

This article deals with 11 skin diseases of dogs and cats, describing the symptoms, discussing the known or possible causes, and outlining any treatments that have been found useful.

The small domesticated animals, particularly the dog and the cat, are subject to a number of different skin affections of a non-parasitic nature. These troublesome and sometimes perplexing afflictions, which are more or less common in dogs and to a lesser extent in cats, include such non-contagious diseases as alopecia, dermatitis, acne, seborrhea, impetigo, urticaria, and eczema, as well as affections due to specific causes such as dermatomycosis, or fungus infection of the skin.

Skin diseases of all types, especially in the dog, are often erroneously referred to by laymen as either mange or eczema. Since each type of skin affection in both dogs and cats usually requires a separate and special treatment, it is highly essential that the nature of the trouble and its cause be definitely determined if possible. Although a tentative diagnosis can be made from the characteristic features in some types of skin disease, it is necessary in most cases to resort to a microscopic examination to determine definitely whether the disease is of a parasitic or non-parasitic nature or whether it is due to fungi. Culture tests are also necessary at times, especially in cats, to determine the presence of ringworm.

When skin affections in dogs and cats become well established or chronic, they are sometimes difficult to cure, requiring persistent and painstaking attention for a long period. Even then results are occasionally unsatisfactory. The best results can be expected when the treatment is under the supervision of a qualified veterinarian with experience in treating small animals.

In the treatment of non-parasitic skin disorders, too much stress should not be placed on external medication. The non-irritating medicinal preparations, such as oils, dusting powders, lotions, and ointments, commonly used on skin affections are merely relief measures to allay itching and promote healing and in most instances do not remove the primary cause of the trouble, which must be done in order to effect a cure.

The causative factors in non-parasitic skin diseases, except ringworm and favus (a specific skin affection due to fungi), are numerous and sometimes obscure.

The appearance and condition of the coat of dogs and cats are influenced to a great extent by the general health of the animal. Disturbances in the general metabolism brought about by infectious conditions, diseases of the digestive, nervous, circulatory, or excretory systems, faulty feeding, and the administration of certain drugs are usually reflected in the skin and hair. Although the skin and hair normally show a marked resistance to ordinary external conditions, certain mechanical, chemical, or temperature influences have an extremely irritating effect, and, together with invasion by infective organisms, play a part in the production of skin affections.

Alopecia (Loss of Hair)

Loss of hair, or alopecia, may be general or localized. A general loss of hair may occur in the normal process of molting. A dog normally sheds its coat once or twice yearly, the old hair being replaced with a new growth in about 6 weeks. Heavy-coated dogs and long-haired breeds that are kept indoors in the winter may shed more or less continuously. The annoyance caused by shedding can be lessened to some extent by daily grooming and keeping the dog outdoors. General shedding may also occur in debilitating diseases, such as distemper, diabetes, and jaundice, and as a result of senility. A localized loss of hair may occur in such skin diseases as mange, ringworm, and eczema, and in infestation by lice or fleas. It is also seen as a result of burns, scalds, chemical irritants, and thyroid deficiency.

Dandruff, or Scurfiness

Dandruff is characterized by the presence of grayish-white scales on the skin or in the hair due to excessive exfoliation (falling off) of the upper layer of the skin. A dry, scaly skin may be caused by the use of strong bath soap, irritating chemical preparations, decreased sebaceous secretion, parasitic infestation, digestive disorder, and deranged secretion of the thyroid gland. Daily grooming to stimulate local circulation and the application of coconut or olive oil to relieve dryness are sometimes beneficial. When loss of hair accompanied by scurfiness is due to thyroid deficiency, the condition may be improved by a course of treatments with thyroid extract.

Dermatitis

Inflammation of the skin (dermatitis) in dogs and cats is usually accompanied by redness (erythema), itching (pruritis), and sometimes loss of hair (alopecia) and the formation of dandruff (scurf). Skin ruptures consisting of papules (pimples), vesicles (blisters), and pustules (purulent papules) may also occur in some forms of dermatitis.

Dermatitis may be local or general and may occur as an acute or subacute inflammation. It may also occur as a symptom during the course of distemper in dogs, or as a secondary symptom in parasitic infestation with tapeworms, hookworms, or heart worms. It is most commonly caused by extremely irritating external influences, such as pressure and rubbing from collars and harness, close clipping, the use of stiff grooming brushes, running through bushes, insect bites (by flies, fleas, bees, or wasps), and lying on hard rough floors. Prolonged exposure to the direct rays of the sun, burning, scalding, and freezing may also produce a form of dermatitis, and the condition may appear after a bath with strong caustic soaps or the application of irritating chemicals to the skin.

Dermatitis is usually characterized by redness of the skin and extreme itching. Repeated scratching, rubbing, and licking of the affected part tend to aggravate the condition. The lesions, or injuries, produced by the scratching and rubbing are frequently invaded by dirt and infective micro-organisms (*Staphylococcus* or *Streptococus*, which often set up a septic dermatitis.

Mild forms of the disease usually clear up in a short time after the cause is determined and eliminated. The application of soothing lotions such as witch hazel or ichthyol ointment to relieve the itching, and dusting with mild antiseptic powders such as boric acid are usually beneficial.

During the fly season a dermatitis of the ears causes much concern to dog owners in many localities. Flies attack the tips of the ears and sometimes the eyelids and corners of the mouth, producing a dermatitis which, if untreated, may become very serious. When it is impractical to confine dogs in screened kennels, this condition can be relieved to some extent by the application of an ointment comprised of 5 per cent of oil of tar in a lanolin base. This serves both as a healing agent and as a fly repellent.

Chronic cases of dermatitis accompanied by a thickening and hardening of the skin with a discharge of serum, formation of crusts, and loss of hair require long and persistent treatment to effect a cure and often terminate in chronic eczema. In persistent cases in which the condition can be ascribed to no external irritant, the animal should be examined for the presence of intestinal parasites. The diet should be checked and altered if necessary to provide a balanced ration.

Eczema

Eczema, which is frequently mistaken for mange or ringworm, is often referred to by laymen as red mange. It is one of the most common skin diseases in dogs but is less prevalent in cats.

The disease is characterized by erythema, the development of papules, vesicles, and pustules, a serous discharge, formation of crusts, intense itching, appearance of scurf, loss of hair, and a marked tendency to become chronic.

Eczema occurs in two forms–as an acute moist condition referred to as weeping eczema, or, more commonly, as a dry chronic condition. In the acute form the development of the disease is rapid.

It is characterized principally by an intense erythema, marked itching, the formation of vesicles, a serous exudate, loss of hair and a glistening. moist appearance of the skin. This type frequently affects long haired dogs.

The chronic type usually starts as a simple dermatitis and slowly develops into chronic eczema. It is characterized by inflammation and eruptions of the skin, intense itching, loss of hair, and formation of scurf, crusts, and scabs. It appears to be more common in coarse- and wire-haired breeds of dogs.

The most common site for the development of eczema is the region around the base of the tail and extending along the back line to the shoulders and neck. The skin around the scrotum or the vulva is also often affected. A moist form of eczema with a brownish discharge often affects the ear canal and the skin between the toes.

The disease is most prevalent during the summer, especially during hot, humid weather. In some dogs it has a tendency to clear up during the winter months, only to reappear during the early spring and summer. On account of its seasonal occurrence it is frequently referred to as summer eczema or periodic eczema.

The different forms of external irritation mentioned as possible causes of dermatitis may also be the primary causative agents in eczema.

A number of other factors, a few of which appear to have some connection with the fact that the disease occurs in summer, have been advanced as possible causative agents:

(1) Allergy–certain foodstuffs, principally those with a high protein content, are believed to produce a reaction in the skin known as allergic eczema;

(2) Hypersensitivity, manifested in some dogs by extreme sensitivity to certain drugs and chemicals;

(3) Photosensitization, a condition that occurs in animals with light skin due to certain sensitizing agents as well as to lack of protective skin pigmentation and producing a mild inflammation or extensive blistering of the skin;

(4) Fungus infections, prevalent principally during the summer;

(5) Flea or chigger infestation, common during the summer;

(6) Environment–for example, confinement in small, hot, poorly ventilated quarters, with little or no exercise;

(7) Faulty feeding, including overfeeding, feeding excessive amounts of proteins or carbohydrates, and vitamin or mineral deficiencies.

General measures for the control of this trouble include reducing the protein or carbohydrate content of the diet, decreasing the food intake of overfed dogs, bathing less frequently, regular brushing and combing to keep the hair and skin clean, keeping affected animals in cool, dry, well-ventilated quarters free from flies and other insects, regular exercise in the cool part of the day, regular evacuation of the bowels and bladder, and keeping the animal free from internal parasites and particularly from such external parasites as fleas, lice, ticks, and harvest mites.

The use of mild lotions, ointments, and dusting powders to allay itching and promote healing is of some value in most cases.

Impetigo

Impetigo is rare in adult dogs but occasionally occurs in puppies. It is characterized by an eruption of small yellow vesicles or pustules which spread rapidly and tend to rupture, discharge a yellow pus, and later form scabs. The abdominal surface and the region inside the thighs are most commonly affected. It may occur as a secondary symptom in intestinal parasitic infestation, distemper, and other infectious diseases. In treating this condition applying a mild antiseptic to affected areas is helpful.

Seborrhea

Seborrhea, commonly known as greasy skin, is due to an excessive secretion of the oil glands of the skin. The condition occurs most frequently in fat, overfed house pets deprived of regular exercise.

The lesions first appear in the region of the ears, neck, and root of the tail and gradually extend to other areas. The hair has an oily appearance and may gradually fall out, and there is usually an unpleasant characteristic odour associated with the malady.

Acne

Acne in dogs and cats, also known as furunculosis or folliculitis, is an inflammation of the hair follicles or the skin glands, with a bacterial invasion resulting in suppuration (discharge of pus). It is characterized by the appearance of pimples or pustules which rupture, discharge pus, and form dry scabs. The condition most frequently affects the skin of the face, particularly the nose and cheeks, but may occur on other parts of the body. As the disease progresses, boils or carbuncles may develop at the site of the original lesions. In the treatment of the condition, good results have been reported following the administration of autogenous bacterins (those made from bacteria isolated from the skin lesions of the affected animal). Local treatment consists in opening the nodules and applying mild antiseptics to the affected parts. The administration of arsenicals internally has also been reported of value in some cases.

Furunculosis in cats frequently follows bites, bruises, and other injuries to the skin. The root of the tail and the back are the regions most commonly affected. The condition has a tendency to spread and become chronic, and surgical treatment is often required to effect a cure.

Lip Ulceration in Cats

Ulceration of the skin of the upper lip is a condition peculiar to cats. It usually becomes chronic and does not respond readily to treatment. Good results are sometimes obtained by treating with iodine preparations. Application of silver nitrate (5 percent) has also been reported to be of some value.

In treating skin affections in cats under no circumstances should soaps or disinfectants containing phenol, creosote, tar, creolin, or naphthol be used, as cats are extremely sensitive to these materials.

Urticaria

Urticaria, also known as nettle rash and hives, is rather uncommon in the dog. It is characterized by the sudden appearance of large blotches or swellings. The eruptions may be found on all parts of the body surface, but sometimes they are confined principally to the head, causing a diffuse swelling of the skin of the face. The exact cause of the disease is not known. Sometimes it is apparently due to external irritation, but in most instances it appears to be the result of an intestinal toxemia, or poisoning brought about by faulty feeding. Allergy has also been advanced as a cause. The course of the disease is usually short. Affected animals recover, and lesions disappear in many instances within a few hours without treatment. Recovery can be hastened by the administration of purgatives.

Ringworm

Ringworm is a communicable disease of the skin occurring in both dogs and cats and readily transmissible to man and some other animals. The disease is caused by specific fungi (chiefly *Microsporon* and *Trichophyton* species), which are somewhat similar to certain ordinary molds. The lesions of ringworm usually appear On the face, head, or legs, but they may occur on any part of the body.

The disease in dogs is characterized by small circular areas of dirty gray or brownish-yellow crusts or scabs partially devoid of hair. As the disease progresses, the lesions increase in size and number and merge to form larger patches covered with crusts containing broken-off hairs. A raw, bleeding surface appears when crusts are removed by scratching or rubbing to relieve itching. In some cases, however, there is little or no itching.

In cats the lesions appear as small, raised, scaly or scabby areas covered by hair, but detectable by running the finger tips over the skin. Microscopic examination and culture tests are necessary for an accurate diagnosis.

If treatment of affected dogs is started early, when only a few lesions are present, the disease can be cured in 5 or 6 weeks. Treatment consists in clipping the hair from around the lesions, removing scabs, and applying tincture of iodine or 5-percent salicylic acid solution two or three times weekly until recovery takes place. Scabs and hair removed during treatment should be burned to destroy the infection. Due precautions should be observed in handling animals affected with ringworm, as this disease is readily transmissible to man and other animals. Isolation of affected animals is essential to prevent the spread of the disease.

Favus

Favus is caused by a fungus known as *Achorion schonleinii*. It occurs principally in young cats and rarely in dogs. The sites most frequently affected are the paws, especially the skin of the toes near the claws, and the head and face. Lesions may occur in other parts of the body.

The disease is characterized by circular yellowish or grayish patches that develop into thick layers of crust of a sticky consistency.

Applications of tincture of iodine, a 5-percent solution of chlorine, or a 5-per cent solution of salicylic acid are of value in treatment. This condition, like ringworm, is contagious to human beings, and affected animals should therefore be isolated and handled with due precautions.

Chapter 11

NUTRITIONAL DISEASES OF DOGS AND CATS

I.P. Earle [1]

[1] *I.P. Earle is Associate Biochemist, Animal Nutrition Division, Bureau of Animal Industry.*

As they occur under practical conditions, nutritional diseases are more likely to be the result of several dietary deficiencies than of any single one. It is well to know the characteristics of single vitamin and mineral deficiencies, however, as a guide to the proper feeding of dogs and cats and an aid to the diagnosis of nutritional diseases.

The ancestors of the dog and cat hunted food for themselves and their young from the plains and the woods. Since they ate the vitamin-rich organs and viscera of their prey and the mineral-rich bones as well as the muscles, they probably suffered from no nutritional deficiencies as long as game was plentiful and they were skillful and lucky as hunters. Their meat diet was probably supplemented occasionally with a few green leaves, and they had free access to sunshine. The descendants of these hardy ancestors for the most part no longer hunt their own food but remain in the kennel, around the house, or in the house and accept the food provided for them by man. The food may be the scraps from the table, or it may be mixture of various products of the slaughterhouse and the mill. In either case the adequacy of the diet largely depends on the care and judgment of the human master.

Some metabolic disturbances in dogs and cats are produced by hereditary defects, but many other conditions of this nature are brought about by a deficiency or unbalance of the nutritional factors required by the animal for maintenance, growth, reproduction, and physical activity. Sometimes nutritional deficiencies are secondary to other conditions which interfere with the proper assimilation and utilization of nutritive factors, but more often they are the direct result of an inadequate supply of the required factors in the diet.

Although many studies have been made of the nutritive requirements of dogs and of the effects of specific deficiencies, little is known concerning the nutritional requirements or nutritional diseases of cats. However, since the dietary habits of the wild members of the cat and dog families are somewhat similar, it is assumed that the two species are probably subject to similar deficiency diseases. This assumption is supported by what scant knowledge is available concerning the nutritional diseases of cats.

The most commonly occurring errors in the diet of domestic pet animals are deficiencies in vitamins, minerals, and proteins of good quality. Except in the case of rickets, a positive diagnosis of which can be made by means of the X-ray, some information concerning the previous diet of the animal is often essential in diagnosing a disease of nutritional origin. The careful investigations of the laboratory have been concerned chiefly with the effects of deficiencies of single factors, whereas the disease conditions resulting in actual practice from dietary deficiencies are more often the result of multiple deficiencies. Also the characteristic effects of specific deficiencies usually occur in combination with non-specific symptoms which may be induced by one or more of several causes. The most common of these non-specific symptoms is the retardation of growth, which may result from simple starvation, inadequate proteins of good quality, deficient or unbalanced calcium or phosphorus, or a deficiency of one or more of several vitamins. Likewise a degeneration of the central and peripheral (outer) nervous system, with resulting incoordination of movements, may occur as result of vitamin A deficiency or of some type of vitamin B deficiency.

Some of the more common diseases which are fairly easily recognized as of nutritional origin when they occur in dogs are discussed here. Although the discussion shows that the use of pure vitamins, either by injection or by addition to the feed, may be of value in the treatment of a disease condition for the immediate relief of symptoms, the use of a well-balanced diet of natural feedstuffs which contain adequate amounts of the essential factors constitutes the most important treatment for deficiency diseases, as well as the best preventive measure.

Rickets

Any disturbance in the mineral metabolism that results in defective or abnormal calcification, or hardening, of growing bones is usually termed rickets. The clinical indications of rickets include lethargy and listlessness, arched neck, crouched stance, knobby and deformed joints, bowed legs, and flabby muscles. The changes characteristic of defective calcification in the young animal are most marked in the zones of growth of the long bones of the legs–at the junction of the end (epiphysis) and shaft–and at the cartilaginous junction of the ribs. At such points there is a cessation of calcification with an excessive production of cartilage and a deposition of fat. In the more advanced stages the entire bone becomes soft and easily deformed or broken. The development of the teeth is also retarded.

The X-ray is a reliable and practical means of diagnosing early rickets and of determining the severity of the disease and the progress of healing. In the dog the characteristic changes are easily recognized, especially in the lower end of the ulna–the large bone of the foreleg-at the joint which corresponds to the wrist joint in man. In the young animal the calcified shaft of the long bone is separated from its more lightly calcified head by a band of uncalcified cartilage. Normally this cartilage grows and is rapidly calcified at the end of the shaft; as the animal matures the cartilage decreases in width and eventually becomes calcified. In the rachitic animal, however, the cartilage continues to grow but is not calcified, thus increasing the width of the uncalcified band. Changes in the normal calcification of bone may be detected by means of the X-ray at a much earlier stage than that at which clinical evidence of rickets appear.

It is now known that rickets may result from a deficiency of calcium, phosphorus, or vitamin D and that it may be prevented and cured, if it is not too advanced, by the inclusion in the diet of adequate amounts of calcium and phosphorus and enough vitamin D to regulate the absorption and assimilation of the minerals.

The dog's requirements for the three factors calcium, phosphorus, and vitamin D have been studied extensively by Morgan and associates (*17, 18, 19, 21, 22*).[2] She has demonstrated that in puppies fed on diets deficient in either calcium or phosphorus severe bone deformities result. The conditions produced by the mineral deficiency can be ameliorated but neither prevented nor cured by vitamin D. She has noted, however, that rickets in dogs is usually of the low-phosphorus type, and has ascribed the condition to a faulty utilization of phosphorus rather than to a deficiency of phosphorus in the diet, since low-phosphorus diets are less likely to be encountered than low-calcium diets. The phosphorus in the cereals which frequently form a large part of the dog's ration is not well utilized by the dog.

There is a wide divergence in the estimates made in different laboratories of the requirements of the dog for vitamin D. The requirements vary with the age of the animal, and apparently with the breed, the amount of sunlight the animal receives, and the ratio of calcium to phosphorus, as well as with the content of calcium and phosphorus, and apparently also a number of other factors in the diet.[3]

It is evident that puppies of the small breeds require far less vitamin D for normal bone development than the large, rapidly growing types with heavy bones. It is also recognized that the requirements of puppies raised indoors are far greater than those of puppies with even limited outdoor life and moderate exposure to sunlight. However, the minimum requirements obviously vary widely with other factors in the ration.

---

2 Italic numbers in parentheses refer to Literature Cited.

3 Arnold and Elvehjem (*1*) found that 5.5 International units of vitamin D per pound of body weight was sufficient to prevent rickets in large-boned puppies on rations containing calcium and phosphorus in a ration of 12 : 1, whereas when the calcium-phosphorus ratio was increased to 2 : 1 this amount of vitamin D was insufficient. It has been reported from Morgan's laboratory (*19*) that with the usual purified ration used there, which has a calcium-phosphorus ratio of 1.7 : 1, 33 units of vitamin D per pound per day is sufficient for Cocker Spaniels, but severe rickets can develop in German Shepherds on this same level. The Fleischmann laboratories (*27*) have reported that although 13 units of vitamin D per pound of body weight per day is sufficient for terrier puppies, growing dogs of large breeds may require more than 123 units of vitamin D per pound of body weight per day. The diet that was used in these studies supplied calcium and phosphorus in a ratio of 2.2 : 1.

Experiments (*19*) with very large doses of irradiated ergosterol equivalent to 4,545 or more International units of vitamin D per pound of body weight per day for several weeks have shown that a condition of hypervitaminosis D–too much vitamin D–can be induced in the dog. This condition is characterized by vomiting, greasy hair, bloody diarrhoea, and deposition of calcium in the arteries and organs. The range between the body requirements and the toxic dose is wide, but the possibility of overdosage should not be overlooked.

The specific treatment of rickets consists in the administration of vitamin D in addition to an adequate supply of calcium and phosphorus. The best sources of vitamin D are fish-liver oils, irradiated ergosterol, irradiated foods, and the action of sunlight on the skin, which enables the animal to manufacture its own vitamin D.

Bonemeal at a level of 1 or 2 per cent of the ration will usually provide sufficient supplementary calcium and phosphorus for puppies of small breeds. Puppies of the larger breeds should have bones and milk in addition. About 0.5 per cent each of calcium and phosphorus (in the mineral form, not as bonemeal) in the diet is probably sufficient, however. Arnold and Elvehjem (*1*) have given as an optimum figure 0.27 per cent for calcium and 0.22 per cent for phosphorus.

Although the requirements of older dogs for calcium and phosphorus and vitamin D are much less than those of young dogs, a condition called osteomalacia, or late rickets, is sometimes observed in grown dogs as a result of the same kinds of deficiencies that cause infantile rickets. In such cases a softening of the bones leads to lameness and deformity.

Tetany of Parturition, or Eclampsia

Eclampsia occurs sometimes in female dogs and cats shortly before, during, or after the delivery of young. It is apparently the result of a calcium deficiency, possibly associated with a vitamin D deficiency. It is most common in females nursing large litters, in which case the demands of the mother for calcium for milk production are heavy. The symptoms vary in severity from nervousness and mild convulsions to severe attacks which may terminate in coma and death. It has been found that the seizures can be controlled by the administration of calcium, and recurrence is prevented by additions of readily utilized calcium and vitamin D to the diet.

Scurvy

Efforts to produce experimental scurvy in the dog with vitamin C-deficient rations have been unsuccessful, and the evidence is that dogs normally synthesize their own vitamin C. Nevertheless, there are occasional reports of a spontaneously occurring condition resembling scurvy which is relieved by the administration of ascorbic acid (vitamin C) or some vitamin C-rich substance such as lemon, juice. Collet (*4*) has described such a condition in young dogs that had been maintained on a diet low in vitamin C. The symptoms observed were a slight anemia, a swelling of the jaw, and signs of pseudoparalysis (a condition resembling paralysis) of the legs. The condition was completely relieved by the administration of lemon or orange juice. Flohil (*9*) also described symptoms resembling those of scurvy which occurred in dogs fed entirely on cooked feeds and which cleared upon the administration of lemon juice. A similar report has been made by Jordan (*15*). Gregoire (*11*) has ascribed a condition in young dogs which he calls Barlow's disease to a vitamin C deficiency in the ration. The animals became anemic, signs of rickets were present, and there was considerable pain on pressure of certain bones near the joints. Although in good condition, the affected animals remained lying down much of the time. He found a lower than normal excretion of vitamin C in the urine of these animals. Some individuals responded to massive doses of ascorbic acid, and others did not. The condition seems to occur only in young animals and appears to result from a failure in vitamin C metabolism, suggesting a failure in the normal functioning of the animal organism in the synthesis of ascorbic acid, the causes of which are not known.

Nutritional Anemias

Anemia is a deficiency in hemoglobin, the oxygen-carrying pigment in the blood. The physiological effects of anemia result from the diminished power of the blood to absorb oxygen and remove carbon dioxide and include an increase in pulse and respiration rates, rapid onset of fatigue with exercise, and general weakness. Even a mild degree of anemia is recognizable by the pale colour of the visiable mucous membranes and by blood examination. Anemias may result from such causes as hemorrhage, internal parasites, chronic infectious diseases, and poisoning, or from a faulty diet. Nutritional anemias occur as a result of diets inadequate in the quantity of the constituents that function in the production of hemoglobin. They are most commonly associated with a deficiency of iron or copper or of the B vitamins, or with long-continued underfeeding of proteins essential for the formation of red blood cells.

Copper itself is not a constituent of the hemoglobin molecule, but it is required by the canine as well as by some other species for the utilization of iron, which is essential in hemoglobin formation. Only minute amounts appear to be needed, however. Potter, Elvehjem, and Hart (24) found that growing dogs made anemic by bleeding responded unfavourably when kept on a diet poor in iron and copper supplemented with 30 milligrams of iron a day, but a rapid regeneration of hemoglobin occurred when the ration was supplemented with 30 milligrams of iron and 4 milligrams of copper. Since copper is required in such small amounts it seems unlikely that the ordinary ration of the dog will ever be deficient in the mineral unless the animal is kept on a diet of milk, which is low in both iron and copper. However, the addition of minute amounts of copper seems advisable when an inorganic iron supplement is used in the treatment of anemia.

An iron deficiency in the dog's ration is not rare, but the iron requirements of the normal dog are amply met by a ration containing as much as 10 per cent of meat scraps or a reasonable amount of fresh meat. The requirements of the bitch are increased during pregnancy, when she may need a more liberal allowance of iron-containing feeds. The normal pup, in common with other sucklings, has at birth a store of iron which is considerably depleted during the suckling period when the principal food is milk. This loss of iron is repaired as soon as iron-containing feeds are added to the diet to supplement the milk. If the pup's diet fails to include feeds that are good sources of iron, an anemia may result which can be cured by correcting the iron deficiency. Feeds of particular value as sources of iron are liver, kidney, red meat, egg yolk, apricots, peaches, and prunes. Small amounts of inorganic iron (iron oxide or iron citrate) may also be used effectively as sources of available iron.

Another type of anemia results from a deficiency of one of the vitamins of the B complex. The production of anemia in dogs maintained on a blacktongue-producing diet (one lacking in part of the B vitamins) was observed by Spies and Dowling (*26*). They effected an immediate correction of the anemic condition by the administration of yeast. They suggested as a possible explanation of the multiplicity of symptoms seen in dogs on this diet that several essential dietary factors are present in that part of the B complex which was lacking in the diet. The more recent work of Fouts, Helmer, and Lepkovsky (*10*), in which an anemia characterized by small, pale red blood cells was produced in dogs maintained on a synthetic diet amply supplemented with other known B factors, has identified the antianemic factor as apparently identical with vitamin B_6 (pyridoxine), the rat antidermatitis factor. Fresh liver, liver concentrates, liver extract, and yeast are most effective in providing the factor B_6, which is required by both pups and older dogs for the maintenance of a normal hemoglobin level.

The treatment of the primary cause of an anemia depends on the factor responsible for the condition, but the treatment of the anemia itself is much the same in all cases. It consists, aside from emergency measures, in the administration in readily available form of ample supplies of the blood-building materials, including proteins of good quality iron, copper, and certain of the B vitamins. Liver, either fresh or dried, is a good source of all these factors. Medicinal supplements of inorganic iron and copper or of liver extract or liver concentrates can sometimes be used to good advantage, together with feeds rich in good proteins and in the B vitamins. Meat diets have been found to be strikingly more efficient in regenerating the blood of dogs after repeated blood depletion than diets rich in carbohydrates or in which the proteins were largely supplied by milk and cereals (*29*).

Vitamin A Deficiency

A diagnosis of vitamin A deficiency in dogs is usually based on symptoms that appear in the advanced stages of the disease, when some animals may fail to recover even when the deficiency is corrected. Probably the most easily recognized symptom is a characteristic disease of the eye called xerophthalmia. Many other conditions less specific and often not so easily recognized as of dietary origin are associated with a deficiency of vitamin A. These include loss of weight, rough coat and scaling skin, in coordination of movements, probably lowered resistance to infections, and, in growing puppies, a stunting of growth.

Frequently the diet supplies almost but not quite enough vitamin A to meet the dog's requirements, and a subacute deficiency extremely difficult to diagnose results. Crimm and Short (*5*) found that the disease in its subacute stages, before the appearance of obvious clinical symptoms, was characterized by a shift in the percentage of immature cells among the white blood cells of a certain type. This they interpreted as indicating a disturbance in the normal formation of white blood cells. Dogs kept for a year on rations in which the vitamin A deficiency was not severe enough to produce loss of weight or xerophthalmia showed changes in the epithelial (surface) cells lining the small bronchial tubes of the lungs as well as changes in the white blood cells.

Experimental work with some other animal species has indicated that one of the earliest symptoms of a vitamin A deficiency is night blindness, or a failure in the adaptability of the eyes to dim light. Although apparently little attention has been given to the effects of vitamin A on the night vision of dogs, it seems likely that the vitamin plays the same role in this species as in the others studied.

While xerophthalmia may develop relatively early in young dogs deprived of sufficient vitamin A, it is indicative of an acute deficiency that develops gradually. First the eyes appear watery and glassy, and the conjunctiva becomes congested. Later the tear ducts become blocked, infection appears, and there is inflammation and edema (watery swelling) of the cornea and finally ulceration. Permanent blindness usually results from xerophthalmia after it has reached the advanced stages of severe degeneration of the cornea. Eye symptoms are usually accompanied by other symptoms of disturbances in the body, such as loss of appetite, unhealthy skin and coat, and a muscular incoordination and weakness that eventually end in paralysis. This condition is the result of the nerve degeneration induced by lack of the vitamin.

Deafness appears to be another manifestation of a deficiency of vitamin A which occurs in young dogs. Mellanby (*16*) reported in 1938 that puppies fed for some months on diets of natural feedstuffs deficient in vitamin A evidenced incoordination in movements, inattentiveness, and deafness. He found in such animals an overgrowth of bone near the brain in such a position as to stretch the auditory nerve, thereby causing it to degenerate. Poor growth and faulty tooth development are also associated with a deficiency of vitamin A in the pup.

Higgins (*14*) has reported the experimental production of urinary stones in dogs deprived of vitamin A. There are occasional reports of the finding of kidney or bladder stones in vitamin-deficient dogs on post mortem examination. It has been shown in some other species that a relationship exists between the formation of urinary stones and vitamin A deficiency, but apparently other factors are also involved. The use of vitamin A therapy in the treatment of urinary stones is a subject for further experimentation.

Fish-liver oil is commonly used as a concentrated source of vitamin A for supplementing the diet as well as for medicinal treatment. Bradfield and Smith (*3*), however, have reported that puppies utilize vitamin A in cod-liver oil, pure carotene in oil, and carotene as it occurs naturally in carrots and other foods equally well as a source of vitamin A in repairing a deficiency. Carotene, however, is probably utilized less economically than true vitamin A for storage in the body. Feeds that are particularly valuable as sources of Vitamin A in the dog's diet are liver, green leaves of vegetables, and alfalfa leaf meal of good quality.

Various estimates of the amount of Vitamin A needed by the dog range from 10 International units to more than 360 per pound of body weight. According to suggestions made by Guilbert, Howell, and Hart (*12*), 80 Units (16 micrograms) of Vitamin A per pound of body weight per day is a good allowance for dogs. Morgan (*19*), however, has recommended an amount in excess of 360 International units per pound of body weight per day. In treating a deficiency very large doses can apparently be given with safety.

Deficiencies of the B Vitamins

Thiamin, or Vitamin B_1, Deficiency

Spontaneous outbreaks of a disease in dogs which closely parallels beriberi in humans have been reported. Symptoms are a loss of appetite, vomiting, either a diarrhoea or constipation, cutaneous edema (watery swelling of the skin), muscular tenderness, and a periodic inability to stand. The symptoms yield rather promptly to injections of thiamin and to the addition to the diet of dried brewers' yeast or some other good source of Vitamin B_1.

The antiberiberi factor (vitamin B_1, or thiamin) is required preformed in the ration for the normal growth of young dogs and the maintenance of health in both young and adults. The earliest and most conspicuous effect of a deficiency is a marked loss of appetite, which occurs in dogs more promptly as a result of thiamin deficiency than of any other vitamin deficiency. In general, the symptoms associated in the dog with a deficiency of vitamin B_1 may be grouped as arising either from the failure of normal functioning of the gastro-intestinal tract, with a marked loss of tone, or from disorders of the nervous system. The appearance of symptoms varies with the severity of the deficiency and undoubtedly with the extent of complications arising from other deficiencies that may result from decreased food consumption or impaired absorption and assimilation. The early stages of the deficiency are marked by loss of appetite, fatigue, nervousness, restlessness, and irritability, whereas the advanced stages are characterized by manifestations of polyneuritis (inflammation of many nerves at once) such as muscular tenderness, incoordination of movements, and paralysis of the hindquarters.

Although degenerative changes in the nerves have often been demonstrated in association with thiamin deficiency, more recent evidence (*8*) shows that the nervous symptoms of uncomplicated thiamin deficiency are not due to any actual break-down of tissues in the nervous system. When degeneration of nerve tissues occurs, it may probably be attributed to deficiencies of vitamin A or of other factors of the B complex. The profound nervous disturbances which occur in an uncomplicated deficiency of thiamin and which respond within a few hours to the administration of thiamin are probably produced by disturbances of nerve metabolism rather than by degenerative changes in the nerve tissues themselves.

Thiamin is believed to have a specific role in the carbohydrate metabolism of nerve tissue. The thiamin requirements of the animal are related directly to the nonfat calories of the diet rather than to body weight; hence diets low in fat and high in carbohydrates require a higher level of thiamin than diets high in fat. Arnold and Elvehjem (*1*) have shown that both growing and mature dogs can be protected from the loss of appetite associated with thiamin deficiency by 360 micrograms, or 120 International units, of thiamin to each pound of a ration low in fat. This supplies 3 to 4.5 units of thiamin per pound of body weight per day for an average-sized mature dog. Therapeutic (medicinal) doses of 10 times this amount or more have been used to give prompt relief from nervous symptoms of thiamin deficiency.

Of the group of B vitamins, thiamin is the most easily destroyed by heat. It has been shown that as much as 80 per cent of the thiamin content may be lost during the canning of dog food. Likewise the processing of meat scrap at high temperatures reduces the thiamin content. Gram byproducts from which the germ and outer covering have been removed, as well as all processed foods, are likely to be low in this vitamin.

Thiamin occurs, along with other members of the B complex, in organ and muscle meats (pork muscle is 7 to 8 times as rich in thiamin as beef muscle), yeast, the germ and outer portions of grains, milk, egg yolk, and most fruits.

Fright Disease

Fright disease is adequately discussed in the article by C.D. Stein. However, since there have been many reports of a response of the condition to a change of ration and other reports of the immediate relief of symptoms with thiamin treatment in cases characterized by the nervous-running-howling-convulsions complex, the possible relation of the condition to a thiamin deficiency should be mentioned here. Patton (23) has recently observed the production of fright disease in dogs fed a certain commercial feed low in vitamin B_1. The nervous condition was relieved within a few hours by thiamin injection. Many attempts have been made to produce the condition on experimental diets low in thiamin, diets low in protein, and diets containing protein denatured by heat. Arnold and Elvehjem (2) succeeded in producing the symptoms with a diet of meat scrap and wheat which had been heated to 392° F., the animals failed to respond to thiamin administration.

Riboflavin Deficiency

Since a deficiency of riboflavin, or vitamin B_2, probably never occurs spontaneously in the diet of the dog except in the presence of deficiencies of other B Vitamins, the specific effects of a riboflavin deficiency alone may never be observed uncomplicated by other factors except in the laboratory. These effects consist, in the early stages, of a variable dermatitis, or skin inflammation, partial loss of appetite, and loss of weight and, in the acute stages, of sudden collapse followed by death unless treatment with riboflavin intervenes. The dermatitis appears first as a reddening of the skin, followed by a dry scaliness. It occurs usually on the chest and abdomen and the inner surfaces of the legs near the body. In the male it involves the scrotum. In the acute stage of the deficiency the animal becomes apathetic, walks with a staggering gait if it walks at all, and evidences a marked weakness. If no treatment is given the animal soon passes into a coma and dies within several hours, apparently from respiratory failure. Sebrell and Onstott (*25*) have described a characteristic yellow mottling of the liver and degenerative changes in the central nervous system in such animals.

The injection of 0.34 milligram of riboflavin per pound of body weight into animals in this collapsed state results in prompt recovery if given in time. Street and Cowgill (*28*) have found that 11.4 micrograms of riboflavin per pound of body weight per day in the ration is sufficient to satisfy the dog's requirements for an extended period.

Riboflavin is widely distributed in plant and animal tissues. It is present in milk, meat, yeast, eggs, and many fruits and vegetables. It occurs in higher concentration in the liver and kidney than in muscle meat. Yeast is an especially rich source. Although it is less sensitive to heat than thiamin, riboflavin is destroyed by high temperatures somewhat above boiling. The content of riboflavin in meat is decreased by frying or roasting.

Blacktongue and Nicotinic Acid

Elvehjem, Madden, Strong, and Woolley (*6*) were the first to report that nicotinic acid will prevent and cure the condition in dogs known as blacktongue. It has recently been shown by Heath, MacQueen, and Spies (*13*) that cats are subject to a similar condition which responds to the same treatment. However, as this disease occurs spontaneously, it is probably the result of a multiple deficiency, since ordinary rations deficient in nicotinic acid are likely to be deficient in other vitamins of the B complex also. The occurrence of blacktongue has been observed most often in those areas of the South where the dog's ration is somewhat similar in character to the diets producing pellagra in man, that is, where the ration consists largely of such products as corn meal, salt pork, cowpeas, and sweetpotatoes.

The onset of typical blacktongue is characterized by lassitude, loss of appetite, and sometimes vomiting. The mouth gives off a characteristic foul odour. The mucous membranes of the cheeks, gums, and tongue are reddened and inflamed, sometimes showing more or less extensive purplish-red areas where the congestion is most marked. The front end of the tongue is most likely to be affected in this way. The inner surfaces of cheeks and lips may even be covered with pustules and ulcers. Constipation is often noted at the onset of the disease, and a diarrhoea develops in the later stages.

If the disease has not progressed too far, recovery may be effected by proper treatment; otherwise, death results. Nicotinic acid or liver extract may be given by injection as an emergency measure. Attention should be given to cleansing the mouth, if this is needed. Aside from these measures, treatment consists in adjustment of the diet to include foods such as fresh liver, dried yeast, beef muscle, wheat germ, eggs, and milk, which are good sources of nicotinic acid and other vitamins of the B complex.

It has been shown that 0.23 milligram of nicotinic acid per pound of body weight per day will cure the symptoms of blacktongue in the dog (7). Half this amount is probably sufficient to give protection against blacktongue, although it will not promote normal growth in young dogs.

Morgan (*20*) has called attention to the possible dangers of administering large amounts of nicotinic acid in the presence of a deficiency of other factors of the B complex. She has observed that dogs receiving purified rations deficient in both nicotinic acid and the so-called filtrate fraction of the B complex suffer a more rapid decline if nicotinic acid alone is administered than if neither factor is given. In the treatment of blacktongue, care should be exercised to avoid bringing about a condition of unbalance among the various B factors by using nicotinic acid alone without including other factors of the B complex.

Deficiencies of Other Factors of the B Complex

The anemia produced by a deficiency of pyridoxin, or vitamin B_6, has already been mentioned.

In addition to thiamin, riboflavin, nicotinic acid, and pyridoxin, dogs require two or more of the remaining factors of the B complex. It has been shown that pantothenic acid is necessary for normal growth and health of the dog, and that filtrate factor W, referred to as the anti-gray-hair factor, is necessary for the maintenance of a healthy condition of the fur and for neuromuscular control. Morgan (*20*) has demonstrated an interrelation between nicotinic acid, pantothenic acid, and the filtrate factor W and has indicated that there may be other factors of the B complex which have a function in canine nutrition. The requirements for pantothenic acid and the factor W are not yet determined.

Literature Cited

(1) ARNOLD, AARON, and ELVEHJEM, C.A. (1939). NUTRITIONAL REQUIREMENTS OF DOGS. Amer. Vet. Med. Assoc. Jour. 95: 187-194, illus.

(2) _____and ELVEHJEM, C.A. (1939). IS RUNNING FITS A DEFICIENCY DISEASE? Amer. Vet. Med. Assoc. Jour. 95: 303-308, illus.

(3) BRADFIELD, DOROTHY and SMITH, MARGARET CAMMACH (1938). THE ABILITY OF THE DOG TO UTILIZE VITAMIN A FROM PLANT AND ANIMAL SOURCES. Amer. Jour. Physiol. 124: 168-173.

(4) COLLET, P. (1935). LA MALADIE DE BARLOW SPONTANEE CHEZ LE CHIEN (SCORBUT INFANTILE). Rev. Vet. [Toulouse] 87: 497-537, illus.

(5) CRIMM, PAUL D., and SHORT, DARWIN M. (1937). VITAMIN A DEFICIENCY IN THE DOG. Amer. Jour. Physiol. 118: 477-482, illus.

(6) ELVEHJEM, C.A., MADDEN, R.J., STRONG, F.M., and WOOLLEY, D.W. (1937). RELATION OF NICOTINIC ACID AND NICTOTINIC ACID AMIDE TO CANINE BLACK TONGUE. Amer Chem. Soc. Jour. 59: 1767-1768.

(7) _____ MADDEN, ROBERT J., STRONG, F.M., and WOOLLEY, D.W. (1938). THE ISOLATION AND IDENTIFICATION OF THE ANTI-BLACK TONGUE FACTOR. Jour. Biol. Chem. 123: 137-149, illus.

(8) ENGEL, R.W., and PHILLIPS, P.H. (1938). THE LACK OF NERVE DEGENERATION IN UNCOMPLICATED VITAMIN B_1 DEFICIENCY IN THE CHICK AND THE RAT. Jour. Nutr. 16: 585-596.

(9) FLOHIL, J. (1933). SCORBUT BIJ HONDEN [SCURVY IN DOG]. Tijdschr. v. Diergeneesk. 60: 633. [In Dutch. English summary, p. 634.]

(10) FOUTS, PAUL J., HELMER, OSCAR M., and LEPKOVSKY, SAMUEL (1940). NUTRITIONAL MICROCYTIC HYPOCHROMIC ANEMIA IN DOGS CURED WITH CRYSTALLINE FACTOR I. Amer. Jour. Med. Sci. 199: 163-166.

(11) GREGOIRE, C. (1938). VITAMIN C AND BARLOW'S DISEASE IN THE DOG. Ann. Med. Vet. 83: 366-371. [Abstract in North Amer: Vet. 21: 164. 1940.]

(12) GUILBERT, H.R., HOWELL, C.E., and HART, G.H. (1940). MINIMUM VITAMIN A AND CAROTENE REQUIREMENTS OF MAMMALIAN SPECIES. Jour. Nutr. 19: 91-103, illus.

(13) HEATH, M.K., MACQUEEN, J.W., and SPIES, T.D. (1940). FELINE PELLAGRA. Science 92: 514.

(14) HIGGINS, C.C. (1936). URINARY LITHIASIS. EXPERIMENTAL PRODUCTION AND SOLUTION WITH CLINICAL APPLICATION AND END-RESULTS. Jour. Urol. 36: 168-177.

(15) JORDAN, MARJORIE G. (1940). A CASE OF VITAMIN C DEFICIENCY. Vet. Jour. 96: 214-215.

(16) MELLANBY, EDWARD (1938). THE EXPERIMENTAL PRODUCTION OF DEAFNESS IN YOUNG ANIMALS BY DIET. Jour. Physiol. 94: 380-398,. illus.

(17) MORGAN, AGNES FAY (1933). EFFECT OF DIET ON RESPONSE TO PARATHYROID EXTRACT AND VITAMIN D. IV. THE EFFECT OF DIETS OF NORMAL CALCIUM AND PHOSPHORUS CONTENT IN DOGS. Amer. Jour. Physiol. 105: 621-634, illus.

(18) _____ (1934). THE EFFECT OF ACID, NEUTRAL, AND BASIC DIETS ON THE CALCIUM AND PHOSPHORUS METABOLISM OF DOGS. Calif. Univ. Publs., Physiol. 8: 61-106, illus.

(19) _____ (1940). DEFICIENCIES AND FALLACIES IN CANINE DIET. North Amer. Vet 21: 476-483.

(20) _____ (1941). THE EFFECT OF IMBALANCE IN THE "FILTRATE FRACTION" OF THE VITAMIN B COMPLEX IN DOGS. Science 93: 261-262.

(21) MORGAN, AGNES FAY, and GARRISON, E. ALTA (1933). THE EFFECT OF DIET ON RESPONSE TO PARATHYROID EXTRACT AND VITAMIN D. II. THE EFFECT OF HIGH CALCIUM-LOW PHOSPHORUS DIETS IN DOGS. Amer. Jour. Physiol. 105: 596-607. illus.

(22) _____ GARRISON, E. ALTA, and HILLS, MARGUERITE J. (1933). THE EFFECT OF DIET ON RESPONSE TO PARATHYROID EXTRACT AND VITAMIN D. III. THE EFEECT OF LOW CALCIUM-HIGH PHOSPHORUS DIETS IN DOGS. Amer. Jour. Physiol. 105: 608-620, illus.

(23) PATTON, JOHN W. (1939). FRIGHT DISEASE AN AVITAMINOSIS. Vet. Med. 34: 372-381, illus.

(24) POTTER, V.R., ELVEHJEM, C.A., and HART, E.B. (1938). ANEMIA STUDIES WITH DOGS. Jour. Biol. Chem. 126: 155-173.

(25) SEBRELL, W.H., and ONSTOTT, R.H. (1938). RIBOFLAVIN DEFICIENCY IN DOGS. U.S. Pub. Health Serv., Pub. Health Rpts. 53: 83-94.

(26) SPIES, TOM D., and DOWLING, ALEXANDER S. (1935). THE EXPERIMENTAL PRODUCTION OF ANEMIA IN DOGS BY MEANS OF A BLACKTONGUE-PRODUCING DIET. Amer. Jour. Physiol. 114: 25-29, illus.

(27) STANDARD BRANDS INCORPORATED (1939). A SYLLABUS ON VITAMIN D AND METHODS OF SUPPLYING IT TO FARM ANIMALS. Vitamin D Digest 1: 37-40.

(28) STREET, HAROLD, R., and COWGILL, GEORGE, R. (1939). ACUTE RIBOFLAVIN DEFCIENCY IN THE DOG. Amer. Jour. Physiol. 125: 323-334.

(29) WHIPPLE, G.H., ROBSCHEIT, F.S., and HOOPER, C.W. (1920). BLOOD REGENERATION FOLLOWING SIMPLE ANEMIA. IV. INFLUENCE OF MEAT, LIVER AND VARIOUS EXTRACTIVES, ALONE OR COMBINED WITH STANDARD DIETS. Amer. Jour. Psysiol. 53: 236-262.

INDEX